Implementing excellence in your health care organization

Implementing excellence in your health care organization

Managing, leading and collaborating

Edited by Rob McSherry and Jerry Warr

Open University Press

Open University Press
McGraw-Hill Education
McGraw-Hill House
Shoppenhangers Road
Maidenhead
Berkshire
England
SL6 2QL

email: enquiries@openup.co.uk
world wide web: www.openup.co.uk

and Two Penn Plaza, New York, NY 10121-2289, USA

First published 2010

A catalogue record of this book is available from the British Library

ISBN-13: 978033523477-6 (pb)   978033523476-9 (hb)
ISBN-10: 033523477-1 (pb)   0335233476-3 (hb)

Library of Congress Cataloging-in-Publication Data
CIP data applied for

Typeset by RefineCatch Limited, Bungay, Suffolk
Printed in Great Britain by Bell and Bain Ltd., Glasgow

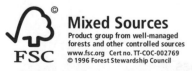

Mixed Sources
Product group from well-managed
forests and other controlled sources
www.fsc.org Cert no. TT-COC-002769
© 1996 Forest Stewardship Council

The McGraw·Hill Companies

Contents

Figures

Tables

Contributors

Claire Brewis is Principal Lecturer/Subject Group Leader in Occupational Therapy at the University of Teesside.

Corrina Dickson is a Research Development Officer at Bournemouth University.

Lee-Ann Fenge is Senior Lecturer in Social Work at Bournemouth University.

Karen Grimwood is Senior Lecturer in Child and Community at the University of Teesside.

Sarah Hean is Senior Lecturer in Research Methods at Bournemouth University.

Vanessa Heaslip is Lecturer in Adult Nursing at Bournemouth University.

Jenny Kell is Principal Lecturer in Service Improvement at the University of Teesside.

Rob McSherry is Professor in Nursing and Practice Development at the University of Teesside.

Mel McSherry is Senior Lecturer in Adult Nursing at the University of Teesside.

Sabi Redwood is Senior Lecturer in Qualitative Research/Ethics at Bournemouth University.

Lisa Smith is National Improvement Lead for National Health Service Improvement in Leicester.

Kevin Stubbings is Modern Matron for Mental Health Services Older People in Teesside.

Jackie Tonkin is Social Worker for Mental Health Services Older People in Teesside.

Katie Tucker is Methodology Developer in Leeds.

Jerry Warr is Reader in Practice Development at Bournemouth University.

Acknowledgements

The editors would like to personally thank all the contributors for the time and effort devoted to preparing the chapters for the book. Without your contributions the book wouldn't be possible. Thank you also to Rachel Crookes (Commissioning Editor, Open University Press) for continued support and requests to meet the deadlines. Finally thank you to our families for the continued support especially when time is precious.

Introduction

It is a pleasure to present book two, *Implementing Excellence in your Health Care Organization: Managing, Leading and Collaborating,* in the 'Excellence in practice development in health and social care' series. The aim of the series of texts is to provide a clearer understanding of what we mean by 'excellence in practice' by providing a practical framework to support health and social care professionals to achieve this within the context of individual, team and/or organizational practice. *What makes an organization 'excellent'?* Organizations are complex concepts embracing cultural, political and personal elements that contribute to their activities, performance and outcomes. Jones (1994: 444) reminds us that 'an organisation is not just a group of people although relationships between people are fundamental to it; it is a social unit deliberately set up to achieve specific goals'. The European Foundation for the Improvement in Living and Working Conditions (2007: 4) imply that a successful organization is interdependent on teamworking, resolving cultural difference and in creating a working environment that fosters and values performance: 'The challenge for companies [indeed health and social care organisations] is to deliver quickly and flexibly new products and services, in order to be able to respond to greater and changing demands for clients'.

Burton et al. (2005) cited by The European Foundation for the Improvement in Living and Working Conditions (2007: 4) argues that for an organization to achieve high performance, the workplace should focus on 'increasing people's influences on the business as well as the impact of process, methods, physical environment, and the technology and tools that enhance their work'.

The aspirations offered by the above embrace issues surrounding dynamics, power, collaboration and effective teamworking. While the title is 'working in health care organizations', the ability to work 'by, through and with' are central components in collective working. Excellence in practice and indeed in oneself is dependent on how efficient and effective an organization is in leading, managing and supporting people and the associated systems and process in maximizing the best possible outcomes and therefore achieving excellence. Building on the introductory nature of book one in our series, this second book explores in detail the key issues and factors that influence the workings of an organization and how these may be addressed through collaborative working and user-focused care. The book is presented in three sections: Part 1: *Working in organizations*; Part 2: *Collaborative working*; and Part 3: *User-focused care*. The emphasis of the text is on demonstrating through real-life application along with the backing of evidence how practice development and associated tools, techniques and methodologies have and can be applied to any health and social care organization to demonstrate and achieve excellence in practice.

What's in the book?

Part 1 on 'Working in organizations' contains three chapters outlining the associated evidence, which can enhance or hinder the provision of excellence within the working organization through exploring:

- shared visioning through teamworking and personal development
- the importance of management and leadership development and styles
- how adopting a whole systems approach to viewing organizational change could be the catalyst for enhancing the quality of the service.

Part 2 on 'Collaborative working' contains three chapters highlighting the importance of multi-professional working and development, integrated teamworking and inhibitors to collaborative working.

Part 3 on 'User focused care' contains four chapters highlighting the reforming agenda and the importance of working in partnership with users and in seeking users' views and their involvement in care. The chapters cover:

- opportunities and challenges surrounding the meaning of user involvement and making this happen
- ethical and governance issues pertaining to user involvement and how these may be addressed.

Furthermore, the many different ways of engaging users and the importance of equity and equality are central to the whole of this text.

The contributors come from a diverse range of health and social care backgrounds and have been selected because of their focus and experience in practice development that allows realistic and practical exemplars from their own profession and disciplines to be presented. The chapters reflect the format of book one by including activities, case studies and suggestions for further reading but they also embrace the individuality and creativity of the contributors and the dynamic nature of practice development.

By adopting this approach we hope you gain valuable insight into how practice development fosters person or people centeredness in striving for excellence in practice development in the working of any health and social care organization. We would personally like to thank all the contributors for their invaluable contribution to support the development of the book and series.

Rob McSherry and Jerry Warr

References

Burton, B. et al. (2005) The high performance work place defined, cited in The European Foundation for the Improvement in Living and Working Conditions (2007) *Teamwork and High Performance Work Organisation*. Available online at www.eurofound.europa.eu/ewco/reports/TN0507TR01/TN0507TR01.pdf (accessed 18 December 2008).

The European Foundation for the Improvement in Living and Working Conditions (2007) *Teamwork and High Performance Work Organisation*. Available online at www.eurofound.europa.eu/ewco/reports/TN0507TR01/TN0507TR01.pdf (accessed 18 December 2008).

Jones L. J. (1994) *The Social Context of Health and Health Work*. Basingstoke: Macmillan.

PART I
Working in organizations

Shared vision through team and professional development

Corrina Dickson and Karen Grimwood

Introduction

> There is no more powerful engine driving an organisation toward excellence and long-range success than an attractive, worthwhile, and achievable vision of the future that is widely shared (Ideabridge, 2002: 1).

Defined as an imagined concept of how an organization should look, shared vision is inspirational, meaningful, motivational and critical in creating organizational change. The first half of this chapter addresses the importance of shared vision in creating organizational change; exploring the relationship between empowerment, ownership and commitment. It documents the role of shared vision in leadership and highlights how this role is critical in preventing coercion and resistance. Two examples from practice are given to demonstrate the role of shared vision in practice development; one documents a failure and the other a success.

The second half of this chapter outlines the role of communication in creating a shared vision. The various components and strategies used in communication are explored: roles, channels, listening skills and techniques. Two exercises are presented to help identify existing skills and areas of improvement in practice. Finally, the (SMCR – source, message, channel and receiver) model (Berlo, 1960) of interpersonal communication is outlined that offers practical elements to consider when communicating shared vision.

Shared vision

> Visions . . . may be said to be the stuff of organizational success, but not if they hold little meaning for people who work in the organization (Tietze et al., 2003: 135).

To create genuine organizational change, a cultural shift needs to occur; 'culture' referring to the continually evolving beliefs, values and behaviour of a group constructed of basic assumptions they share (Schein, 2004). In order for changes to be incorporated into a culture, followers need to be sufficiently involved in the process as they must recognize the need for change (Klein, 2004) and connecting with followers' values and beliefs is therefore critical in demonstrating that change is necessary. Leaders must create a shared vision that encompasses the goals, values and cultural beliefs of followers in order to inspire and motivate (Tietze et al., 2003), to provide organizational direction and to align followers to move in the same direction (Thornberry, 2006).

Followers are considerably more likely to support what they have helped to create (Vogt, 2008) and therefore they do not simply want to hear a leader's vision, but instead how their own aspirations will be achieved (Kouzes and Posner, 2007: 18). Followers must believe that their ideas can have an impact on the leader's vision for the organization in order for them to partake in changes (Farmer et al., 1998).

When initiating any major change within an organization, creating a vision is critical as it provides followers with a 'map' to interpret actions undertaken as part of the change process and enables them to understand how the actions relate to the future of the group (Tietze et al., 2003). It is essential as vision binds leaders and followers in action, inspiring them to work together to create change; it is through shared vision (and not rules and procedures) that leaders gain genuine commitment from and control over their followers (Halbestram, 2006). When followers are inspired by a shared vision, they excel and help create change because they also see it as necessary; vision therefore fosters genuine commitment rather than compliance to change (Senge, 1990).

Change initiatives often do not succeed because leaders fail to create a shared vision; instead, creating a strategy or mission statement (Burnes, 2004). Shared vision is an achievable imagined concept of how an organization should look (Burnes, 2004), a shared dream of the future based on the reality of how the organization is at its very best (Vogt, 2008). A shared vision needs to be inspiring, meaningful, memorable and vivid. This is difficult to sum- marize into a one or two-line statement and therefore the most effective way to disseminate vision is through a visual image as 'words alone rarely carry long-term meanings for people unless the message behind them can be visualized' (Thornberry, 2006: 32).

A successful vision includes the group's purpose or reason for being, the cultural beliefs and values of stakeholders, the ultimate mission of the organization and the groups' goals and objectives (Thornberry, 2006). So, for example, if a health care organization wished to initiate practice devel- opment, its purpose would be to provide excellence in practice for patients through a multidisciplinary empowered team approach. The cultural beliefs and values would have to be adjusted as the hierarchy of the organiza- tion needs to support the empowerment of practitioners and patients. The mission, goals and objectives must be a bold statement that could be achieved if followed by the whole team such as 'We excel in practice through our work as an emancipated multidisciplinary health care team'.

This would then be depicted into a visual picture illustrating members of the multidisciplinary team chatting together and excellence in care being demonstrated.

A shared vision will be continually re-evaluated, as goals will inevitably change making the process of creating a shared vision a never-ending process (Hodgkinson, 2002). It is a process and not a destination within itself (Thornberry, 2006).

Shared vision and empowerment

Empowerment is central to the concept of practice development and also shared vision as followers need to feel empowered in order to have influence over creating a shared vision, as it is through a shared vision they can become further empowered (Halbestram, 2006). Empowerment is an individual's feeling of having a sense of personal power and the freedom to use this power, developed through identification with the values and ideals of a vision and through the freedom to act and be creative (Lashley, 2001). Empowerment occurs when leaders communicate their vision to followers who are given the opportunity to explore the ideas presented and internalize the new values (Marquis and Huston, 2006).

Voluntary involvement in change is critical for empowering strategies to be successful (Marquis and Huston, 2006), but the rhetoric of 'handing down power' is often preached while suggestions made by staff are ignored (Senior, 2002). Organizational change is most often instigated by hierarchically senior members of a group that means there is a temptation to use hierarchical power to force compliance, leading only to resistance (Seibert et al., 2003) as the following quote reflects. 'Even though hegemonic practices proclaim the value of autonomy, the use of velvet language of participation, involvement or empowerment, they are ideologically engineered to benefit only the interests and goals of managers and owners' (Hatch and Cunliffe, 2006: 267). Instead, a shift in cultural value and belief systems must occur to dissipate restricting hierarchical boundaries.

Organizational stories reflect the extent to which leaders adjust values and beliefs. Positive experiences told through these stories help strengthen a shared vision (Vogt, 2008) while negative experiences recounted as organizational stories cause resistance to changes (Hatch and Cunliffe, 2006: 267). If leaders do not connect with their followers' values, goals and beliefs, changes forced on their followers will incite resistance expressed through the creation and recounting of negative organizational stories. Organizational stories exist to highlight important events in an organization's lifespan such as any major change initiative. They are known by a large number of people within the organization (Johnson and Scholes, 2006). Organizational stories are attempts to recreate reality poetically; not 'facts' but rather individual products of experience (Gabriel, 2000) and extremely powerful in creating unanimous resistance to change. It is for this reason that creating a vision that genuinely connects to followers' beliefs and values is critical.

To create empowerment leaders must hand over a portion of their control (Klein and Lundin, 1999); forcing participation incites only compliance, not commitment that can spark resistance strategies (Seibert et al., 2003). Followers resist partaking in change initiatives because either they do not understand or agree with the reasoning for it; therefore creating a vision that is shared between leaders and followers is essential. When followers help create the goal of the change, understand their role within it and how the proposed actions will help achieve it, they will participate. Making a vision a shared reality 'means involving the hearts and minds of those who have to execute and deliver . . . these are not the people at the top of the organization, but those at the bottom' (Harvey Jones, 1998: 65).

Shared vision in leadership

Creating a shared vision is one of the most important tasks a leader has (Farmer et al., 1998) and it is an essential skill particularly within the transformational leadership and shared leadership approaches (Marquis and Huston, 2006) – both advocated in practice development literature. A transformational leadership approach highlights the importance of providing followers with a compelling vision or sense of purpose and communicating vision clearly. Transformational leaders positively transform and empower their followers (Halbestram, 2006) by addressing their needs, focusing on values and emotions (Northouse, 2004), building a trusting relationship (Rickards and Clark, 2006) and encouraging followers to accomplish more than is expected of them (Kirby, 2000). They shape imagery in the minds of their followers through the articulation of their vision and their actions (Rickards and Clark, 2006) and continually remind their staff of what is important in their role and in a change initiative through shared vision and inspiration (Goffee and Jones, 2006).

The shared leadership approach involves a number of leaders and shared vision is used as their binding force. Disagreements over tasks and changes between the leaders can occur in the early stages of this approach as when a group forms each member has a unique, individual picture of the organization at its best (Tietze et al., 2003). As the group work together to share their own visions and develop an understanding of one another's values, goals and needs, the creation of a vision between them occurs (Schein, 2004). Once established it becomes a collective mental reality the group can imagine achieving and then work with their followers to refine (Senge, 1990). Commitment to a shared vision is more critical in shared leadership than any other leadership approach as no permanent single leader exists (Burke et al., 2003), meaning the power and control tactics ordinarily utilized cannot be used (Seibert et al., 2003). The success of the group is dependent entirely on

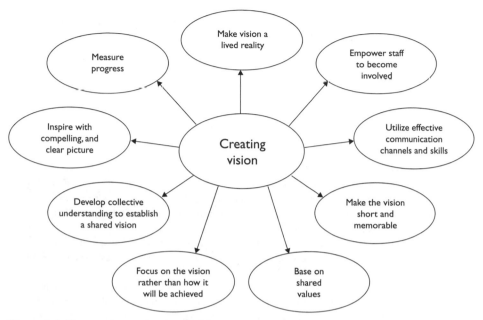

Figure 1.1 Elements in creating shared vision

each individual member's commitment to their shared vision (Rickards and Clark, 2006).

This chapter has so far outlined the importance of shared vision in organizational change, empowering change strategies and related leadership approaches. Figure 1.1 summarizes the elements explored that are necessary to create a successful vision.

The following two examples from practice are based on the experience of the authors and highlight how shared vision can be created in practice both successfully and unsuccessfully. The remainder of the chapter focuses on the role of communication when creating a successful shared vision.

Example from practice 1.1   Failure to create shared vision as a group

Dickson (2008) documents the failure of one multidisciplinary health care team to become an accredited practice development unit (PDU) under the scheme offered at Bournemouth University. The scheme promotes shared vision as an essential element in successfully implementing practice development. However, the hierarchically senior core group of practitioners leading the change created a shared vision only among themselves, and not with the rest of the staff they worked with. The core group wished to unify two wards of staff in order to weed out the poor performers and while never verbalized the staff were aware of this. The core group used practice development accreditation as a method to impose changes on their staff, under the guise of a shared vision.

Why was the shared vision not successful?

There were a number of factors that made this an unsuccessful example of creating shared vision:

* The core group did not involve staff in creating a shared vision, but rather imposed their own vision on staff and as a result the staff refused to participate in activities related to the new vision.
* The core group were also reluctant to listen to any ideas from staff as this did not fit in with their vision for the new structure, leaving staff feeling disempowered 'They pay no attention . . . if you come up with an idea and put that idea forward, you can guarantee that it won't happen' (Dickson, 2008: 205).
* The staff were consciously resistant as a result of being forced into participating in activities related to the new vision 'There will be resistance from all of us' (Dickson, 2008: 183).
* The failure to create a genuine shared vision and internalize new values associated with practice development meant the core group did not recognize that forcing staff to participate is a direct violation of this approach and the accreditation attempt failed.

Example from practice 1.2   Successfully creating a shared vision as a group

Similar to the scheme offered at Bournemouth University, the Excellence in Practice Accreditation Scheme (EPAS) at Teesside University advocates creating a shared vision as a critical element of creating successful development in practice (McSherry et al., 2003). This example discusses how this is facilitated. Groups undertaking the EPAS are introduced to the concept of shared vision and to ensure full understanding appropriate language is used with the aim to instigate participation.

Strategies used for creating the vision

Through the use of a facilitator, individually and collectively the group were asked to 'brainstorm' ideas in order to identify their views on what the service should ideally look like. This was achieved through developing an open and honest atmosphere and through the use of various sources of communication; written, oral or electronic, formal and informal. Thus, there was a sense of involvement and empowerment and ownership of the ideas. Even some group members who were initially disinterested in creating a shared vision became engaged and it became possible to articulate the various skills and attitudes of each member of the group. Once these appropriate communication methods were established group members captured their ideas on paper and submitted this shared vision for further discussion and review before it was adopted as a key feature of the unit's development towards accreditation.

What lessons can be learnt from the above experiences?

It is critical that all group members are involved in order for it to be a success and actions in practice must match the vision as failure to do so can act as a barrier (Bell et al., 2008). It is recommended that time in practice is assigned for regular team meetings with the leader(s) of the accreditation attempt to ensure the vision remains clear, relevant and shared. The EPAS and Bournemouth University PDU Scheme are examples of facilitated approaches that promote excellence in practice guided by the shared vision of the group, communicated through a range of appropriate channels.

Communicating shared vision

Creating a shared vision is a difficult enterprise in itself; the practical logistics of the number of people involved, cultural values of language and dialect and gender must all be taken into account when considering communication. Without effective communication a shared vision will fail to be developed or be embraced; communication is pivotal to unlocking a shared vision. Mixed messages can be inadvertently given verbally and symbolically and the need to develop pertinent and valuable communication skills in addition to inter-personal, self-awareness and reflective skills is therefore essential.

There are multiple aspects to effective communication and the remainder of this chapter explores key elements of this. Communication models, methods and frameworks are outlined as well as processes used to develop, apply and reflect on these to enhance professional development, practice and to communicate shared vision of the future.

Communication refers to interactions where messages are both sent and received, through which we present ourselves and interpret the other (Deux and Wrightsman, 1984). Communication is also the process humans use to define reality itself (Stewart, 1999); more than a one-way transfer of information, it is a technique in which minds interact and new ideas emerge to create new understandings (Wiecha and Pollard, 2004: 6).

Communicating effectively involves verbal interactions but also a vast array of other symbols, such as body language, representations and images (as most face-to-face communication is non-verbal, Birdwhistell, 1970), which are used to transfer and develop ideas (McQuail, 1984). Communication is a process 'by which information, meanings and feelings are shared by persons through the exchange of verbal and non-verbal messages' (Brooks and Heath, 1985: 11); these verbal and non-verbal elements containing multiple sub-components. Verbal messages are expressed through tone, volume, dialect and jargon and non-verbal messages are expressed through written words and body language, proximity, eye contact and symbols such as visual images, emblems and clothing. The following sections illustrate the importance of verbal and non-verbal communication in developing a shared vision.

Once appropriate communication methods have been established, group members can engage in creating shared vision facilitated through effective leadership. It is critical that all group members are involved in order for it to be a success and actions in practice must match the vision as failure to do so can act as a barrier (Bell et al., 2008). It is recommended time in practice is assigned for regular team meetings with the leader(s) of the accreditation attempt to ensure the vision remains clear, relevant and shared. The EPAS and Bournemouth University PDU Scheme incites excellence in practice guided by the shared vision of the group, communicated through a range of appropriate channels.

Communicating as a group

To develop a shared vision, effective communication is the key, as in order to fully understand the message being communicated, an understanding of the dynamics and relationships members of a group have must be gained. Consideration must be given to individual group members' 'conceptual filters' (Ellis and Fisher, 1994) – beliefs, values, motives and personalities – as successful teams are defined by good communication streams and clearly defined roles (Jones, 1997).

It is critical for leaders to communicate shared vision but also to help develop this as a group; failure to do this was demonstrated in Example from practice 1.1. Leaders need to have effective communication skills and interpersonal skills (Choi and Pak, 2007) in order to disseminate information, to make each group member feel valued, to maintain constant effective communication (Mencher, 2008) and to empower followers allowing them to engage in the vision as if it was their own (Marquis and Huston, 2006).

Effective communication

Communication channels are effective through both formal and informal structures. Formal communication follows structured pathways where informal channels transfer messages rapidly with a relatively high degree of accuracy within an organization that extend downwards, upwards or horizontally (Northouse and Northouse, 1985). The direction of communication should be based on the requirement of the situation (Hudson, 2004) and in all cases it is essential that each group member is listened to, allowing them to feel valued, making engagement more likely and enabling empowerment to occur.

One of the most effective communication skills is listening; this is not a passive skill but one that requires active hard work (Stanton, 1990). The use of non-verbal communication can be used to reinforce listening; a simple nod of the head, eye contact or a smile are all non-verbal signs that demonstrate listening. Skills and techniques to demonstrate active listening in developing shared vision include effective body language, reflective listening and paraphrasing, asking clarifying questions and to make astute content-to-process shifts 'which enables the listener to hear the many layers of thoughts and feelings that lie beneath the surface of what is being said out loud' (Boesky, 2005).

Traditional communication methods also have an effective role in discussing ideas as part of creating a shared vision; regularly scheduled meetings, reports and memos are all useful but must be used appropriately to meet the group's needs. Group members who are based outside of the practice environment benefit if efficient communication systems (telephone, mobile phone, e-mail, videoconferencing) are established, thereby enhancing communication within the entire group. However, barriers must be set allowing group members to have easy access to each other without encroaching on personal space. While a range of effective communication tools exist, they are supplemental rather than a substitution for face-to-face communication as it is only through this method that non-verbal communication techniques can demonstrate active listening (Mencher, 2008).

While a whole host of tools are accessible to communicate a shared vision, whenever possible communication within a group should be face to face. This should take place without distraction and the valuable resource of time should be negotiated when important information is being communicated; for example, group meetings to discuss shared vision and impart information, within a given time frame, in a suitable environment, free from interruptions and distractions. All team members need to be allowed to communication their ideas, feelings and aspirations to other team members.

Communication of a shared vision is initiated from the leader, who has the vision, to other members of the team. The communication needs to be a two-way process in order that the team members, the followers, feel their ideas are contributing to the vision; hence, the vision then is taken on board as a shared vision by the team.

Communication models

Science always simplifies; its aim is not to reproduce the reality in all its complexity, but only to formulate what is essential for understanding, prediction, or control. That a model is simpler than the subject-matter being inquired into is as much a virtue as a fault, and is, in any case, inevitable (Kaplan, 1964: 280).

This section outlines the simplest and most influential message-centered model of our time (Gronbeck et al., 2004) to illustrate key considerations for creating a shared vision in practice. Berlo (1960) created the SMCR to depict the underlying structure of the communication process. It is acknowledged that models are used to impose pattern on the intricate and complex process of communication (Northouse and Northouse, 1985) and that the subject of communication is multifaceted and complicated. Berlo (1960) recognized interpersonal communication as a complex, mutually interactive and often subtle process between human beings and so developed the SMCR model to help explain this.

As illustrated in Figure 1.2 the first stage of the SMRC model of communication is the 'source'. This is the generator of the message that takes the form of oral, written, electronic or symbolic communication. The source in our shared vision is the leader communicating the 'message', which is the central element, as this is the transmission of ideas; a shared vision. These notions are linked by 'encoding' that refers to psycholinguistic difficulties of

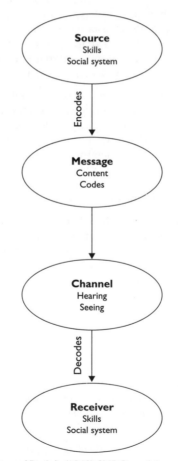

Figure 1.2 Interpretation of Berlo's (1960) SMRC model

translating thoughts into words and symbols. 'Channel' refers to the non-verbal aspects of communication; hearing, seeing, touching. Finally, the model highlights the role of the 'receiver'; the targets of the communication in this example would be the team players who possess the communication skills, attitudes, knowledge, social systems and cultural aspects needed to understand the message being presented by the leader. These notions are linked by 'decoding' that refers to psycholinguistic difficulties in deciphering words or symbols into more understandable terms. These four elements are pertinent in any communication process and all four must be used to enable a group to work together; communicating through various effective channels to the receiver, linking those with differing value belief systems together as a group.

Conclusion

This chapter demonstrated the role of shared vision in practice; achieved through outlining its necessity in organizational change, transformational and shared leadership and its ability to incite ownership, empowerment and commitment. The examples from practice demonstrated how a failure to create a shared vision can be catastrophic, inciting coercion and resistance but also how utilizing effective communication techniques can create a successful shared vision, strengthening teamwork to create change. Finally, Berlo's (1960) SMCR model was outlined in order to demonstrate key aspects to consider when communicating shared vision as a group.

As this chapter has demonstrated, creating a shared vision in practice is a complex and often difficult process. It requires excellent interpersonal and facilitation skills as it necessitates the adjustment of underlying values and beliefs to incite commitment, energy and motivation to change. Failure to create shared vision incites compliance at best, resistance at worst. Successfully creating a shared vision however incites commitment, ownership, and empowerment and can help groups produce amazing results in practice.

Key points

- Shared vision is critical to creating cultural change.
- Vision is an achievable, imagined concept of how an organization should look.
- Leaders must create a shared vision that encompasses the goals, values and cultural beliefs of followers.
- Followers must recognize the need for change and be involved in the process.
- Failing to create shared vision can incite resistance and coercion.
- Vision must be inspiring, meaningful and memorable and is best communicated visually.
- Effective communication is pivotal to unlocking shared vision.

- Communication through both language and symbols, through formal and informal methods, is imperative.
- Consideration must be given to individual 'conceptual filters'.
- The SMCR model provides a guide to key aspects of communication.
- Creating vision is a continual process.

Further reading

Alpert, H., Goldman, A., Kilroy, C. and Pike, A. (1992) Toward an understanding of collaboration, *Nursing Clinics of North America*, 27: 47–59.

Birchall, J.L. (1997) Patient-focused care: anatomy of a failure, *Holistic Nursing Practice*, 11: 17–20.

Bull, P. (1983) *Body Movement and Interpersonal Communication*. Chichester: Wiley and Sons.

Burnard, P. and Gill, P. (2008) *Culture, Communication and Nursing*. Edinburgh: Pearson Education Ltd.

Eagan, G. (1973) *Face to Face, the Small-group Experience and Interpersonal Growth*. Pacific Grove, CA: Brooks/Cole Publishing Company.

Eigeles, D. (2003) Facilitating shared vision in the organization, *Journal of European Industrial Training*, 27(5): 208–19.

Fagan, C.M. (1992) Collaboration between nurses and physicians: no longer a choice, *Academic Medicine*, 67(5): 295–303.

Hoe, S.L. (2007) *Shared vision: a development tool for organizational learning development and learning in organisations*, 21(4): 12–13.

Kikoski, J.F. (1993) Effective communication in the intranational workplace: models for public sector managers and theorists, *Public Administration Quarterly*, 17(1): 84–95.

Pike, A. (1991) Moral outrage and moral discourse in nurse-physician collaboration, *Journal of Professional Nursing*, 7: 351–63.

Qvertveit, J. (1993) *Coordinating Community Care: Multidisciplinary Teams and Care Management*. Buckingham: Open University Press.

Scherer, K. and Ekman, P. (1982) *Handbook of Methods in Nonverbal Behaviour Research*. Cambridge: Cambridge University Press.

Trueman, M. (1991) Collaboration: a right and responsibility of professional practice, *Critical Care Nurse*, 11: 70–2.

Shannon, C. and Weaver, W. (1949) *The Mathematical Theory of Communication*. Champaign, IL: University of Illinois Press.

Swansburg, R.C. (1995) *Nursing Staff Development: A Component of Human Resource Development*. Boston, MA: Jones and Bartlett Publishers.

Useful links

Boesky, J. (2005) Active & Effective Listening Skills. Available online at www.johnboesky.com/article_activelistening.html (accessed 27 November 2008).

IdeaBridge (2002) Creating a compelling vision. Available online at www.jobfunctions.bnet.com/abstract.aspx?docid=162657&tag=rel.res2 (accessed 27 November 2008).

References

Bell, K. Kinder, T. and Huby, G. (2008) What comes around goes around: on the language and practice of 'integration' in Health and Social Care in Scotland, *Journal of Integrated Care*, 16(4): 40–8.

Berlo, D.K. (1960) *The Process of Communication*. New York: Holt, Rinehart and Winston.

Birdwhistell, R. (1970) *Kinesics and Context: Essays on Body Motion Communication*. Philadelphia, PA: University of Pennsylvania Press.

Boesky, J. (2005) Active and effective listening skills. Available online at www.johnboesky.com/article_activelistening.html (accessed 27 November 2008).

Brooks, W. and Heath, R. (1985) *Speech Communication*. Dubuque, IA: W.C. Brown.

Burke, C.S., Fiore, S.M. and Salas, E. (2003) The role of shared cognition in enabling shared leadership and team adaptability, in C.L. Pearce and J.A. Conger (eds) *Shared Leadership: Reframing the Hows and Whys of Leadership*. Thousand Oaks, CA: Sage Publications, pp. 103–22.

Burnes, B. (2004) *Managing Change*, 4th edn. Essex: Pearson Education Limited.

Choi, B. and Pak, A. (2007) Clinical investigator medical, 30(6): 224–32.

Deux, K. and Wrightsman, L. (1984) *Social Psychology in the 1980s*, 4th edn. Monterey, CA.: Brooks/Cole Publishing Company.

Dickson, C. (2008) 'I bet you wish you'd picked a different group': an ethnographic study of practice development accreditation. Unpublished PhD thesis.

Ellis, D.G. and Fisher, B.A. (1994) *Small Group Decision Making: Communication and the Group Process*, 4th edn. New York: McGraw-Hill.

Farmer, B.A., Slater, J.W. and Wright, K.S. (1998) The role of communication in achieving shared vision under new organizational leadership, *Journal of Public Relations Research*, 4: 219–35.

Gronbeck, B.E., Ehninger, D. and Monroe, A.H. (2004) *Principles of Public Speaking*. Boston, MA: Allyn & Bacon.

Gabriel, Y. (2000) *Storytelling in Organizations*. Oxford: Oxford University Press.

Goffee, R. and Jones, G. (2006) Followership: it's personal, too, in W.E. Rosenbach and R.L. Taylor (eds) *Contemporary Issues in Leadership*, 6th edn. Boulder, CO: Westview Press, pp. 127–8.

Halbestram, D. (2006) The greatness that cannot be taught, in W.E. Rosenbach and R.L. Taylor (eds) *Contemporary Issues in Leadership*, 6th edn. Boulder, CO: Westview Press, pp. 81–6.

Harvey Jones, J. (1998) *Making it Happen*. London: Fontana.

Hatch, M.J. and Cunliffe, A. (2006) *Organization Theory: Modern, Symbolic and Postmodern Perspectives*, 2nd edn. Oxford: Oxford University Press.

Hudson, B. (2004) Whole systems working: a discussion paper for the integrated care network. London: Integrated Care Network.

Hodgkinson, M. (2002) A shared strategic vision: dream or reality? *The Learning Organization*, 9(2): 89–95.

IdeaBridge (2002) *Creating a Compelling Vision*. Available online at www.jobfunctions.bnet.com/abstract.aspx?docid=162657&tag=rel.res2 (accessed 27 November 2008).

Johnson, G. and Scholes, K. (2006) *Exploring Corporate Strategy*, 7th edn. London: Prentice Hall.

Jones, R. (1997) Multidisciplinary collaboration: conceptual development as a foundation for patient-focused care, *Holistic Nursing Practice*, 11: 8–16.

Kaplan, A. (1964) *The Conduct of Inquiry: Methodology for Behavioral Science*. San Francisco, CA: Chandler.

Kirby, J. (2000) Assessed for success . . . nurse-led rheumatology ward . . . practice development unit accreditation, *Nursing Times*, 96(28): 42.

Klein, J.A. (2004) *True Change: How Outsiders on the Inside Get Things Done in Organizations*. San Francisco, CA: John Wiley & Sons, Inc.

Klein, R.L. and Lundin, I.S. (1999) *Managing Change in the Workplace: A 12-step Program for Success*. New York: HNB Publishing.

Kouzes, J. and Posner, B. (2007) Shared vision: get excited about the future, *Leadership Excellence*, 24(6): 18.

Lashley, C. (2001) *Empowerment: HR Strategies for Service Excellence*. Oxford: Butterworth Heinemann.

Marquis, B.L. and Huston, C.J. (2006) *Leadership Roles and Management Functions in Nursing: Theory and Application*, 5th edn. Philadelphia, PA: Lippincott Williams & Wilkins.

Mencher, M. (2008) *Building a Great Team*. Available online at www.gamasutra.com/view/feature. . ./building_a_great_game_team_.php?. . .1 (accessed 26 March 2010).

McSherry, R. Kell, J. and Mudd, D. (2003) Best practice using excellence in practice accredidation scheme, *British Journal of Nursing*, 12(10): 623–9.

McQuail, D. (1984) *Communication, Aspects of Modern Sociology*, 2nd edn. New York: Longman.

Northouse, P.G. and Northouse, L. (1985) *Health Communication: A Handbook for Health Professionals*. Englewood Cliffs, NJ: Prentice-Hall.

Rickards, T. and Clark, M. (2006) *Dilemmas of Leadership*. London: Routledge.

Schein, E.H. (2004) *Organizational Culture and Leadership*, 3rd edn. San Francisco, CA: Jossey-Bass.

Seibert, S.E., Sparrowe, R.T. and Liden, R.C. (2003) A group exchange structure approach to leadership in groups, in C.L. Pearce, and J.A. Conger, (eds) *Shared Leadership: Reframing the How's and Why's of Leadership*. Thousand Oaks, CA: Sage Publications, pp. 173–92.

Senior, B. (2002) *Organisational Change*, 2nd edn. London: Prentice Hall.

Stanton, T.K. (1990) Service-learning: groping towards a definition, in J.C. Kendall and Associates (eds) *Combining Service and Learning: A Resource Book for Community and Public Service*, Volume 1, Raleigh, NC: National Society for Internships and Experiental Education.

Senge, P. (1990) *The Fifth Discipline: The Art and Practice of the Learning Organization*. New York: Doubleday.

Stewart, J. (1999) Introduction to interpersonal communication, in J. Stewart (ed.) *Bridges not Walla: A Book About Interpersoanl Communication*, 7th edn. Boston, MA: McGraw-Hill.

Thornberry, N. (2006) A view about 'vision', in W.E. Rosenbach and R.L. Taylor (eds) *Contemporary Issues in Leadership*, 6th edn. Boulder, CO: Westview Press, pp. 31–44.

Tietze, S., Cohen, L. and Musson, G. (2003) *Understanding Organizations through Language*. London: Sage Publications.

Vogt, J.W. (2008) Grounded visioning: a quick way to create shared visions, *Nonprofit World*, 26(4): 12–14.

Wiecha, J. and Pollard, T. (2004) The interdisciplinary eHealth team: chronic care for the future, *Journal of Medical Internet Research*, 6(3): e22.

2 | Leadership and change management

Mel McSherry, Lisa Smith and Jenny Kell

Introduction

This chapter briefly outlines the drivers for effective leadership by offering a detailed account of what the key terms and phrases mean. An application of the theoretical concepts to practice is made to help to make the principles of leadership meaningful. The latter is achieved by exploring the key characteristics and qualities associated with leadership required to innovate and change practice. Furthermore, leadership is discussed alongside change management theory and practical aspects are offered. The context for leadership and change are reviewed within the organizational culture.

Background to leadership

Drivers for leadership development include a plethora of Department of Health (DoH) documents published since the early 2000s; for example, Making a Difference (DoH, 1999), National Health Service (NHS) Plan (DoH, 2000a), NHS Action Plan Guide (DoH, 2001), NHS Improvement Plan (DoH, 2004a), Meeting the Challenge (DoH, 2000b), Making the Change (DoH, 2001), National Standards, Local Action (DoH, 2004b) Managing for Excellence (DoH, 2002). In social care there has been the Leadership and Management Strategy for Social Care (DoH, 2004c). Indeed, effective clinical leadership has been identified by the government as central to the modernization programme. According to the DoH (2001) '. . . anyone working in the NHS, regardless of their position, grade, qualification or place of work, may be a leader or agent of change and improvement'.

↻ Activity 2.1 Reflective questions

Many well-known leaders have their roots in conflict; they have taken control of a crisis, made decisions, have a vision of what can be done and can communicate it and fill others with enthusiasm. The quality of leadership is arguably central to the survival of groups and organizations. There have been many great leaders. Some leaders are known worldwide, some known nationally, some locally and some personally.

To support you in focusing on the importance of leadership within practice reflect on the above statement and your own experiences to date and note down your responses to the following questions.

- So what is leadership?
- What do you think the concept of leadership is about?
- What do you need to be a leader?
- Are the terms 'leader' and 'manager' interchangeable?
- Think of a leader you know.
- What made them a leader?
- Were they effective?
- What made them effective?

Read on and compare your notes with the content of the chapter.

More recently the Darzi report (DoH, 2008) emphasizes development of high-quality leadership by clinicians and the Leadership Council has been established to analyse gaps in the current NHS leadership approach and develop strategies deal with the findings.

So what is leadership?

At its most elemental and practical level, 'leadership is letting people know their own value and potential so that they can identify this for themselves' (Covey, 2004: 55). The qualities of an effective leader are that they are able to manage themselves well, need to be credible and be a good role model. They should have the skills to commit to a purpose outside themselves and to want to achieve something for the organization. Effective leaders build their competence and focus their efforts for maximum impact, while recognizing their own limitations. They are recognized as being courageous, honest and credible. To lead from the front, a leader has to stick their neck out first. Leaders are often said to have charisma but what does that actually mean? It could be that they have a memorable impact on people and influence others to the extent of arousing devotion. According to Leigh (2008), when achieving a strong impact you are not merely present but actually convey a strong positive presence. Charismatic people communicate their message effectively in terms of clarity of purpose, strength of passion and message content. By sharing passion and enthusiasm, effective leaders engage and help convince people to follow their lead. Leaders may be seen to be confident and this confidence often conveys power that influences and affects other people's thoughts, feelings and behaviour. Being externally confident might dictate what you expect you want to happen! Leaders will often mirror this (Leigh, 2008).

Leadership vision

As already suggested in Chapter 1, a vision is a picture of the future state of the organization; it is the outcome to aim for. The vision should describe a desirable future in a way that conveys meaning and inspiration to others. However, a compelling vision must be vivid, exciting and consistent (Gallo, 2007). Kotter (1996) suggests that without a good vision, a clever strategy or logical plan can rarely inspire the kind of action needed to produce major change. So, leadership is the ability to identify a vision and convey it to others. Leaders are expected to provide vision and inspiration, set goals, motivate, supervise and develop teamworkers. They are concerned with sustaining enthusiasm and willing commitment from staff to do the work that needs to be done. Vision plays a key role in producing useful change by helping to direct, align and inspire actions on the part of large numbers of people (Kotter, 1996). Unfortunately, few leaders communicate meaning, hope and optimism and fail to create an emotional connection with their employees, customers and colleagues (Gallo, 2007). Gallo (2007: 57) also suggests that as a leader you should 'be able to communicate the vision vividly so that others want to be part of the scheme with you'. However, this might be a difficult proposition for clinical leaders working within set boundaries. However, the NHS Institute for Innovation and Improvement (2005) suggests that the vision should be shared by all and be an aim for perfection as aiming for anything less implies that it would be acceptable to deliver care below the agreed standard.

Leadership qualities

Kouzes and Posner (1995) suggest that there are fundamental practices associated with leadership and attempt to offer practical guidance to facilitate demonstration of leadership behaviours. To 'model the way' means never asking someone to do something that you would not do yourself. You have to be open and honest and have firm beliefs and values. This will also ensure a degree of credibility within your clinical team and maintain consistent approaches. Furthermore, effective leaders should 'inspire a shared vision'; this is about having a dream of what could be, and an absolute and total belief in the dream. Leaders who are confident in their ability can make extraordinary things happen. The leader should be able to connect with the followers and be able to speak the same language, understanding their dreams, hopes, aspirations, visions and values.

Kouzes and Posner (1995) go on to state that effective leaders 'challenge the process' and become pioneers that will step into the unknown and become early adopters of innovation. They search for opportunities to innovate. These leaders 'enable others to act' and leadership is seen as a team effort. A simple test is to see if the leader uses the word 'we'; most leaders use 'we' three times more than 'I'. They build trust and make it possible for others to do good work and allow others to feel a sense of personal power and ownership. Finally, effective leaders 'encourage the heart' showing appreciation for people's contributions. It is about linking rewards with performance in an authentic way from the heart. In a clinical context this may be seen as the leader sharing the vision with the team and celebrating small successes as they occur. This also means rewarding individuals who have taken the lead in different aspects of the challenge.

In a similar vein, Covey (1992) offers 7 habits of highly effective people and suggests that leaders should be proactive; this is about being self-aware. Behaviour is a function of decisions, not conditions. You choose how you respond to a stimulus. If you are being provoked, you choose how to respond! There is a difference between being reactive and being proactive. You need to recognize that you have a circle of influence and develop skills to expand your influence within the circle.

Covey (1992) recommends that we begin with the end in mind and asks you to imagine your own funeral. What do you want people to say about you? It is about exploring your personal values and writing a personal mission statement. He encourages you to look at the principles that govern your actions. In putting 'first things first' we explore time management and making priorities. Here the issue of delegation is addressed and distinction is made between urgent and important tasks. To think win-win requires what Covey (1992) refers to as 'interdependence' and mutual respect; these are seen as essential ingredients for success. As adults we should seek to move from dependence to independence to interdependence where the consideration for others is high and personal courage is evident.

Covey (1992) asks that we seek first to understand and he asks that we diagnose before we prescribe. This means gaining a full and comprehensive insight into a situation before attempting to challenge or change the situation. When the leader understands the other person, he or she may then attempt to be understood. Creative cooperation (synergizing) is about creating a high level of communication; the important thing is to ensure that the synergy is positive but being careful to include people with a different perspective so that you do not work exclusively with like-minded people. Covey (1992) states that we need to 'sharpen the saw', a term to express self-renewal. A man sawing down trees needs to take time out to sharpen the saw otherwise the saw becomes blunt and it will take twice as long to achieve the outcome. If he is constantly too busy he will become less productive. In health and social care terms this might be recognized as burnout of staff who continually work under pressure.

Leadership, teamwork and motivation

Leadership is not behaviours and techniques, but a state of being according to Quinn (2004). Leadership is about influencing and without followers there can be no leaders. What would cause someone to follow others? Followers must accept that the leader will produce meaningful change that is in the interests of all the parties. A leader can rarely realize organizational potential alone. It takes team work to turn a vision into reality (Gallo, 2007). Selling the vision is about making it relevant to the team (Gallo, 2007). 'People tend to modify behaviour only when they feel that it is in their own interests as defined by their own values' (Goldsmith and Reiter, 2007: 59). People will always ask 'What's in it for me?' and effective leaders will be able to sell the benefits. Enthusiasm and vision are important but all the passion and mission in the world will not make up for lack of empathy (Gallo, 2007). The key to selling yourself and your ideas, your vision and values is not to announce them but to get others to embrace them and share ownership with the leader (Gallo, 2007).

There is a difference between an achiever and a leader; people become achievers because of the focus on themselves, their career, their performance, their needs and their progress. Leaders are truly great when they shift the focus from themselves onto others (Goldsmith and Reiter, 2007). Effective leaders will praise people and emotionally invest in them. People are rarely overappreciated, but very often underappreciated. People connect with people and not things (Gallo, 2007). As a leader it is imperative to believe in people's ability to succeed and set high expectations. To bring out the best in people, effective leaders will believe only the best about them. A leader needs to lift the tone and genuinely believe in people's ability to succeed. By setting challenging goals and targets, leaders will set high standards and aspirations for the team to strive to achieve (Locke, 1976). People want to live up to what is expected of them (Gladwell, 2000) and it is important to always see tomorrow with optimism. The language and words used should reflect hope, potential and possibility. The opposite of a leader is not a follower, it is a pessimist. In motivational terms, in a sports game players will put themselves where the ball is going to be and not where it has been (Gallo, 2007)! Military leaders know that motivation is contagious; if one person is fired up it rubs off on the next person and the next. Once everyone on the team shares the excitement, they all perform better together (Gallo, 2007). Great leaders tell a powerful, memorable, actionable story (Gallo, 2007).

Types of leadership

There have been several theories of leadership developed and a brief overview will help place the theory to the practical setting. Theories of leadership briefly provided are as follows: great man theory, trait theory, contingency theory, situational leadership theory, transactional leadership theory, transformational leadership, impoverished or laissez-faire, authoritarian or autocratic leaders and democratic leaders.

Great man theory

In the great man theory, the right to lead was viewed as a birthright. Great leaders are born with the natural ability to lead, influence and direct others.

It was in the blood to lead. Only those possessing these qualities were leaders, other people who try to lead are challengers who are seen as opponents or traitors. It was assumed that leaders cannot be developed! Leadership was not seen as a skill that could be taught or coached (Wedderburn Tate, 1999).

Trait theory

The trait theory is based on an assumption that a leader has a set of personal characteristics that include being active, adaptive, assertive and bold. These traits also include being compassionate, concerned and confident. Characteristics of a leader are also thought to be constructive, energetic, engaged, expressive, factual, flexible, grounded, hopeful, humble, independent, integrated, involved, mindful, open, optimistic, principled, questioning, realistic, reflective, responsible, secure, self-disciplined, spontaneous, strong and visionary (Quinn, 2004). The trait approach suggests that leadership exists as an attribute of a personality. However, there are difficulties with the trait theory; for example, early researchers thought that the same traits would work anywhere. Imagine the leadership qualities needed in a cardiac arrest situation compared to a rehabilitation setting. This theory raises questions around what would happen if some traits were missing. Do you need all the same qualities all the time? Another criticism of this theory is that these attributes are often associated with masculine qualities.

Style theory

Style theories are based on an assumption that style matters most. This may be 'task-centred', which is a structured approach, and may be perceived as more efficient, or 'person-centred', which is a supporting approach and could be perceived as more effective.

Contingency theory

Contingency theory suggests that no one style is best but depends on the circumstances. The leadership style needs to fit the expectations of those being led and be consistent with the task in hand (Adair, 1986).

Situational leadership theory

Situational leadership is not vertical or fixed; the emphasis is more about team work. It is possible to make the mistake of overestimating the importance of character traits and underestimating the importance of the situation within the context. Psychologists call this tendency the 'functional attribution error' (FAE) and it occurs as we are more attuned to personal cues than contextual ones (Gladwell, 2000). Blanchard and Hersey (1977) began to examine the context in which leadership occurred; they considered environment and context. Leadership may change within a group depending on the situation and group dynamics. For example, if a soldier, builder and farmer were on a deserted island who would be the leader?

- Soldier, to fight off natives – life saving.
- Builder, erect housing for shelter and comfort – life saving
- Farmer, to sort out land and animals for food – life saving.

Indeed, the solider, builder and farmer all have equal importance. So, can the same leader operate successfully in radically different situations? Does the leader change when the context changes? The answer is based on the leader–member relations and power needed to complete the task.

Transactional leadership theory

Transactional leadership is where followers give loyalty because they get something in return. The leader will reward or punish using a carrot and stick approach. There is an exchange of rewards for compliance within a process of reciprocal influence between the leader and followers; both parties bargain for mutual benefits. This can be seen as manipulative but some people will be happy with the 'rules' of transactions. Most work contracts are based on this principle (Burnes, 1996).

Transformational leadership

Transformational leadership may occur during times of concentrated change, when a new kind of leadership emerges. The leader inspires others to share a vision and followers think differently and change things because they want to. The old value system and hierarchical structure is inadequate. The transformational leader has good insight and seeks to appeal to their follower's better nature to move forward (Burnes, 1996).

Impoverished or laissez-faire leaders

Impoverished or laissez-faire leaders do not lead; they do as little as possible. They are concerned about neither the task nor the people. It is not clear that this person knows what is happening and followers are left to get on with things. This person might assume that their leadership role is based on rank or status in the organization.

Authoritarian or autocratic leaders

Authoritarian or autocratic leaders like to be in charge, they do not like to be questioned and expect that people will do as they are told. Followers might not have any say and are not valued but the work gets done. These leaders use policies, rules and blame and creativity becomes stifled. This style could be highly effective in a task-oriented workplace.

Democratic leaders

Democratic leaders use a style that assumes individuals are motivated by internal forces and use follower participation and majority rule to get tasks completed (Sullivan and Decker, 2009).

Activity 2.2 Leadership traits

Think about some of the examples given above in relation to leadership traits. What different traits have you seen used in different settings?

Read on and compare your notes with the content of the chapter.

Leadership support for the follower

Depending on the context of the setting, the follower might require different styles of support from the leader. For example, in a clinical emergency situation, the team might need clear instruction or direction to complete a task (phone 2222 and ask for the crash team to come to the department). This instruction is highly directive with little support at this time. Consider the needs of a new member of the clinical team; they might require a mentor to give direction or instruction and support to learn new skills for the first few months. Alternatively, in an area where the workload can be emotionally demanding, such as hospice care, the team members might not need direction if they understand their role and workload, but they would need to work in a highly supportive environment to manage emotional challenges. Other settings could have routine care delivery patterns where members know what to do and need little support to function.

What do we mean by clinical leadership?

The NHS Plan (DoH, 2000a) acknowledged that leadership must be evident at all levels of the NHS by both clinical and non-clinical staff if improvements are to be achieved. An authoritarian approach will not facilitate effective change and development. Of course there are difference care settings and organizational differences and contexts must be considered. For example, a highly technical intensive care facility will contrast with a service provided by social services for young adults with learning disabilities in a residential setting. The type and style of leadership will be different as will be the person taking a leadership role. Indeed, it may not be one person leading a team, and Quinn (2004) suggests that the function of leadership is to produce more leaders, not followers. Collaborative working and inter-professional approaches cannot be underestimated. Again, the type and style of the multi-professional team will reflect the type of care setting. Recently, developments have been made to include service users and carers in some operational team structures. Furthermore, it has been suggested that some service users should take a key leadership role in helping to shape service delivery. While this is evident in mental health services, the principles might be applied to other care and treatment services.

⟳ Activity 2.3 Clinical leadership in action

You are the staff nurse in charge of the ward working with an inexperienced junior team. A patient unexpectedly collapses on his bed while you are in the room attending to another patient on your own. When you try to get a response the patient fails to answer; you suspect that he is in cardiac arrest.

Discuss the leadership style you might adopt to manage this situation. Identify the theory from the review of literature sheets and be prepared to state why you have selected this theory type.

- What is your role in this situation?
- What are you trying to achieve?
- List the skills needed by a leader in this situation.
- State exactly what it is that you want the 'followers' to do.
- How will you allocate tasks to the followers?
- What is the role of the followers?
- Discuss the needs that the followers have at different times during the task.
- How might you measure your effectiveness as a leader in this situation?

Having outlined what leadership is and associated qualities and theories along with why and how leadership is associated with enhancing practice, it is important to illustrate the association of leadership with change and improvement.

Change or improvement?

The term 'improvement' is frequently used in contemporary health and social care to describe a range of modernization initiatives. Alternative terms include change management, quality management, and service improvement and service redesign (NHS Institute for Innovation and Improvement, 2005). We will use the term 'change' to encompass these concepts. Change is described as 'a dynamic process by which an alteration is brought about that makes a distinct difference' (Grohar-Murray and Dicroce, 2002: 251). There are of course different types of change such as chaos, unscheduled and reactive change. For the purpose of this chapter, the emphasis will be on planned changed. Planned change can be defined as 'using valid knowledge in a deliberate and collaborative way to improve the operations of human systems' (Marquis and Huston, 1998: 68). The term 'change agent' is used to describe 'a person responsible for changing the target system'. To be effective they should be familiar with the target system and the process of change. The change agent may be as follows.

External – brought in from an external source to impose or facilitate change.
Internal – a senior management figure or someone with successful change project management experience.
Formal – may be directive in approach with a given remit.
Informal – this could be anyone from the team with a good idea.

Source: Buchanan and Huczynski (1997)

The skills of an effective change agent according to Hayes (2002: 19) are as follows:

- communication
- leadership
- teamworking
- confrontational skills
- negotiation
- motivation
- manage relationships.

Based on the works of Hayes (2002), effective communication by the change agent is vital; the change agent must get the right people around the table and make their roles clear. It is essential that the change agent, when making key decisions, needs to be diplomatically positioned so that people are not alienated or left to feel undervalued. It is important to establish the common language of the group. Key stakeholders in the group will include the person who has the management responsibility for the project as a whole. This person must ensure completion on time to an acceptable standard. There may be a person whose agreement is absolutely necessary and may be involved in legal or financial elements of the project. The decider could be a person who has the ultimate decision-making authority and could be the senior manager.

Targets of change

Targets of change is the focus for the change and can be anything including policy change or implementation, procedure and systems change but ultimately it is the person or group who has to change. Three possible targets areas for change are: *knowledge* (awareness raising or developing existing knowledge); *attitude* (affective learning) and *behaviour* of people (compliance to policy/procedures). The leadership role in managing change involves three main responsibilities: achieving the task, building and maintaining the team and development of the individual (Menix, 2000). However, for leaders to manage change requires an awareness of change styles as highlighted in Table 2.1.

Table 2.1 Three change styles

Originators	Pragmatists	Conservers
Future orientated insights that drive change	Encourage cooperation to find solutions	Work well within existing structure
Catalysts for change	Adapt past experience to solve current problems	Consistent and reliable with strong follow-through ability
May overlook relevant details or impact on existing structure	May be too willing to compromise	May delay action and discourage innovation

Having illustrated how leadership can support change and the various change styles, it is important to highlight the models of change.

Models of change

There are numerous models of change. Models of change are often classified by the amount of resistance predicted. To illustrate this in practice, the section highlights the rational model, the forcing model and the coercive model.

The rational model

The rational model is useful when the least amount of power is needed by the change agent and there is no strategy needed to overcome resistance. It is based on the belief that people would change if they knew a better way to achieve a goal. This model works well when a group is motivated and simply needs guidance to make a change; for example, the need to change comes from them. Success depends on compatibility with existing values, trial ability, complexity of change and observable results. The consequence of implementing the change will be team adoption or rejection of the change initiative.

The forcing model

The forcing model is useful when more power is needed by the change agent. The method is to use leverage to get others to change. The objective is to align the change target with established authority. Questions that the change agent should ask include:

Is my authority firmly established?

Is the legitimacy of my directives clear?

Am I capable and willing to impose sanctions?

Is there a clear performance–reward linkage?

Am I controlling the information flow?

Am I controlling the design of the context?

Are the people complying?

Source: Quinn (2004)

When more power is needed by the change agent, Lewin's (1999) three-stage model might be used. Unfreezing is the first stage and this requires identification of driving and restraining forces and once known involves disconfirmation, inducement of guilt and anxiety *but* providing psychological safety, which increases driving forces. The second stage is moving that involves giving information that is needed to implement change, encouraging new behaviour, allowing practice and experimentation, being supportive, allowing opportunities to vent feelings, providing positive feedback with open communication, being enthusiastic, involving staff and educating. The third stage, refreezing, is about continuing to support staff until the change becomes second nature. This model assumes good relationships between change agent and target system and a democratic approach to leadership.

The coercive model

The coercive model might be used when most power is needed; therefore, an authoritarian approach to change that assumes resistance will be substantial. It is often used when more participatory, democratic approaches have failed. Those who use this approach according to Hamilton (1996) enter a win–lose situation and must have enough power to overcome all resistance. It comes with a 'do it or else suffer the consequences' approach.

C Activity 2.4 **Integrating leadership and change management**

You have been told by your line manager that the sickness absence in the department is not acceptable and that your area has the highest incidence of absence in the Trust. You are instructed to implement the Trust sickness absence management protocol.

1 Select a suitable leadership model/philosophy to ensure that you achieve the outcome.
2 Discuss the leadership style you might adopt to manage this situation.
3 Identify the theory from the review of literature and be prepared to state why you have selected this type of leadership style.

Key questions:

1 What is your role in this situation?
2 What are you trying to achieve?
3 How will you achieve this task?
4 How important is this task?
5 List the skills needed by a leader in this situation.
6 What is the role of the followers?
7 Are there any methods you could use to ensure compliance with Trust policy?
8 How might you measure your leadership of this situation?

C Activity 2.5 **Integrating leadership and change management**

You are a new senior lead and you have been asked by your line manager to ensure that all staff have mandatory training updates and that evidence is available to demonstrate this. There are no current records of what training has been undertaken previously.

Discuss the leadership style you might adopt to manage this situation. Identify the theory from the review of literature and be prepared to state why you have selected this theory type.

• What is your role in this situation?
• What are you trying to achieve?
• How will you achieve this task?
• How important is this task?
• List the skills needed by a leader in this situation.
• State exactly what it is that you want the 'followers' to do.
• How will you ensure that the followers attend the training?
• What is the role of the followers?
• Are there any methods you could use to ensure compliance?
• How might you measure your effectiveness as a leader in this situation?

Organizational change

There are numerous theories and models of change: Weisbord's six-box model, Bridges' transitions model and Conner's four roles in implementing change theory (Shapiro, 2004). The tipping point model recognizes that a leader or change agent needs to create contagious commitment through people embracing change. This model suggests that change will only be embraced when enough people sign up the new initiative and that change is a process that evolves over time. Change happens when people change and each person's commitment to organizational change can be contagious. Under the right conditions contagiousness can spread through the organization. This model suggests that people flow between accepting and resisting the change. Levers are designed to encourage contacts between advocates for the change and people who are apathetic about the change. Mass exposure to the change is needed to gain compliance and by recruiting advocates, resistance will diminish. Shapiro (2004) identifies four types of people (or pools) who can influence change:

- **Advocates** – experienced in change and believe it will make a difference.
- **Incubators** – think about the change, not sure that it will help.
- **Apathetic** – not heard of the change or simply do not care. If they ignore the change and it will go away.
- **Resisters** – challenge the change or covertly undermine the change.

The key to successful change implementation lies in understanding why people or organizations resist change, and what exactly the process is to overcome inertia and identify the leadership style required to drive the process in a healthy way. This means more than just good management (Kotter, 1996). Leaders who are fired up about what they do generate excitement in others. Inspiration begins internally and it is only after you identify what you are truly passionate about will you be in a position to motivate others (Gallo, 2007). Effective change agents shape processes to support the organization achieving its goals (Moss Kanter, 1989). Leaders tend to be restless for change, impatient for progress and dissatisfied with the status quo (Gallo, 2007). Great leaders know how to make ambitious goals look doable (Kotter, 1996). Consequently, leadership requires energy, enthusiasm and excitement and this in turn ensures influence. Enthusiasm is infectious and separates average performers from extraordinary leaders (Gallo, 2007).

Effective leaders are not afraid of taking calculated risks. They show this when they have the courage to challenge the status quo, express their point of view, stand up for their beliefs in the face of opposition and deal with any resulting conflict. They can accept alternative views without being defensive and usually make full use of physical expression (Leigh, 2008). The best leaders have passion, commitment and enthusiasm in what they do – if they can transmit their emotion then they will go further in influencing others (Leigh, 2008).

Leadership is a set of processes that creates organizations in the first place and adapts them to significantly changing circumstances. Leadership defines what the future should look like and inspires followers to make it happen despite the obstacles (Kotter, 1996). According to Kotter (1996) successful transformation is 70–90 per cent leadership and only 10–30 per cent management. 'While managers might do what they think needs to be done, growth leaders tend to prioritize and do what needs to be done' (Little, 2008: 77).

Emotional responses to change

We all need to feel that we are doing something worthwhile. We need to feel emotionally fulfilled (Gallo, 2007). The best performing groups are often managed by people with genuine concern for their employees' well-being. Change involves an extremely important component – emotional commitment. All change is a kind of death and all growth requires that we go through a form of depression (Peck, 1987 cited in McConnell, 1998). Perlman and Takacs (1990) describe 10 emotional stages related to change, similar to the grieving process and they suggest action to deal with each stage.

1 People affected by change should have a hand in shaping the change.
2 The nature of the change should be understood by those involved.
3 Ideally it should pose no threat to income or job security.
4 Success of the change initiative is more likely to follow other successful minor changes.
5 The change should be carefully planned.
6 Those affected by the change should have a share in the benefits it brings.
7 People involved should have had relevant training for the new task.
8 It is important that change agents show empathy.
9 There should be effective communication
10 Participate to ensure that there will be a high degree of acceptance by those affected by the change regardless of position or rank.

Resistance to change

Resistance to change occurs when there is misunderstanding and lack of trust in the initiative. Different assessments of need might be made by the change agent and other people involved or expected to implement the change. Parochial self-interest by any member of the team may foster resistance while some people show a low tolerance for change (Kotter and Schlesinger, 1979 cited in Hayes, 2002). Methods for handling resistance include involvement, education and communication for those affected. The change agent should be facilitative and supportive. All people involved should be encouraged to participate and demonstrate involvement. All aspects of the change should be negotiated until agreement is reached. It is important to avoid manipulation and co-optation and implicit and explicit coercion (Kotter and Schlesinger, 1979 cited in Buchanan and Huczynski, 1997). Effective handling of resistance usually involves more than one method. This can be influenced by the personal strengths and limitations of the change agent, such as leadership style, knowledge and skills. There should be a realistic appraisal of the situation and a clear strategy devised. A time span should be set and a speed at which the change must be implemented; patience might be required for long-term goals.

Other reasons for changes that fail are shown in Figure 2.1:

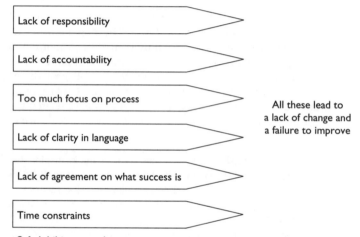

Figure 2.1 Inhibitors to change

Successful proactive change is where people or teams choose to change. Being proactive means taking the initiative and requires good leadership skills. This means focusing on the 'real' problem and solving priorities immediately to invest in the long term. It needs commitment of staff and must be 'controlled' so that forward planning aligns to organizational goals. Being reactive is often seen as being 'managed' and responding to demands. The change agent needs to keep mindful of long-term changes in the environment. Often 'imposed' change, with little consultation, may not take the sensitivity of the people concerned into account. Often, imposed change deals with 'symptoms' and is seen as typical 'crisis management'.

In clinical situations it is important that a process for supporting major organizational change is utilized (Table 2.2). It is also imperative that the above process includes really listening to colleagues and service users at the outset and throughout the process. Without colleagues and service user engagement the change will be seen to be enforced without genuine involvement.

For some people remaining in a stagnant state could be like 'slow death'. The alternative could be deep change and for this we need to come out of the

Table 2.2 Kotter's eight-stage process supporting organizational change

1 establish a sense of urgency
2 create a guiding coalition – with the power to lead change
3 develop a vision and strategy
4 communicate the vision
5 empower broad based action – getting rid of obstacles, changing systems/structures
6 generating short term wins – plan for visible improvements in performance
7 consolidate gains and produce more change
8 anchoring new approaches in the culture

Source: Kotter (1996)

comfort zone and become more purpose-centred and ask the right questions (Quinn, 2004). Rogers (1995), in the diffusion model, identifies reactions to change and suggests that people might be innovators, early adopters, early majority, late majority or laggards. Rogers (1995) found that people's willingness to accept innovation was normally distributed, forming a familiar bell curve. Innovators and early adopters are more willing to adopt innovation. The majority is divided into the early majority, which accepts innovation more easily, and the late majority, who wait until the innovation is almost a new standard before they adopt it. The laggards are the last to embrace a novel approach or technology.

Indeed, change requires personal choice (Quinn, 2004); you cannot just rely on commitment and willpower to change. We live in a dynamic world and work within organizations that have to cope with changing external environments; therefore, 'change' is inevitably always going to pose us a challenge. The way we personally grow in these situations is our choice, but indisputably 'transformation' is always a requirement; how we rise to this depends on our own 'personal state' of self-leadership. Transformation requires sacrifice, dedication and creativity, none of which usually comes with coercion (Kotter, 1996). No matter how capable or dedicated the staff head, guiding coalitions without strong line leadership never seems to achieve the power that is required to overcome what are often massive sources of inertia (Kotter, 1996).

The following criteria are useful for assessing advantages and disadvantages of implementing change. The change

- must be technically feasible
- should be potentially acceptable to all parties
- should be attractive to those whose cooperation is needed
- should be seen as relevant – meeting a need or solving a problem
- should suggest a state of affairs accepted as an improvement
- should be as easy as possible for people to achieve.

When we 'choose' to change we are more likely to be committed. When we do what we 'have' to do we are more likely to be compliant. People need to make the choice. So, how do we make people 'want' to change (Goldsmith and

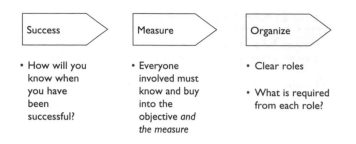

No buy in to the objective and its measure means that the change we seek will simply become a process without result, activity with no output.

Figure 2.2 Organizing for success

Reiter, 2007)? A way to organize for success as highlighted in Figure 2.2. is to involve and inform staff of their role and responsibility within the change. The message is simply short and stark. No involvement and engagement means process without results.

Achieving excellent leadership in practice

According to research presented in 'Diagnosing and Changing Organisational Culture' (Cameron and Quinn, 2006), the style of leadership needs to match the cultural type of the organization. A clan culture with its inherent collaborative orientation requires the leader to be a facilitator, mentor and team builder; within an adhocracy organization where the orientation is primarily creative, the leader style required is innovative, entrepreneurial and visionary; within hierarchical organizations where things are far more controlling, the leader must be predominantly a coordinator, a monitor and an organizer. Finally, in a market culture organization, the leader principally must be a competitor, hard driver and a producer. The highest performing leaders have developed capabilities in all areas (Denison et al., 1995).

Organizational culture

The currency of leadership has been said to be attention. Staff see what the leader does and what attention is given to; this may be the usual topic for discussion (NHS Institute for Innovation and Improvement 2005). According to Covey (2004), 'organizations are made up of people who have relationships and who share a common purpose and each organizational culture is unique, shaped by the values and beliefs of those who inhabit it'. As the organization evolves and takes shape, culture works to coordinate and control behaviour, action and decision-making within the organization. Many organizations are full of potential and promise but they need true parenting, not just caretaking. They need true leadership, not simply management. Individuals in organizations yearn for leaders they can trust and in turn follow (Little, 2008). Culture reflects not just the explicit written rules of the organization but also the unwritten, subconscious, intangible assumptions and beliefs that shape the organizational behaviour and are manifested in all facets of day-to-day life (Graetz et al., 2002). Some examples of the culture include the leadership style; for example, is there empowerment or command and control by senior staff? The language and dress code might reflect the culture – formal or casual?

Communication strategies can also reflect the culture by being one-way or two-way, open and upfront or closed and carefully guarded. The organizational structure might be tall or flat, simple or complex, rigid or fluid, flexible and adaptive. Furthermore, the people that the organization regards as heroes and winners along with the basis of competitive success should be congruent to the organizational aims. For example, do teams work on an individualistic or collective philosophy and how cooperative are individuals in sharing resources for the success of the organization?

There are three layers of corporate culture; artefacts that are observable, such as architecture, office layout, dress code, behaviour patterns, language and documents. This could also be seen in mission statements, directorate objectives and group strategies. A second layer is the values and beliefs of the organization, such as the espoused values and beliefs regarding teamwork, customer service and risk-taking. These may differ to values in action. The third layer is the assumptions held by the team; this is the real core of the culture. The assumptions are often hidden, invisible, and difficult to explain and identify. Assumptions are extremely difficult to change. Management styles are often a reflection of values, beliefs and the situation.

Support for leaders

Leaders need support in the form of mentors/coaches (Quinn, 2004). However, mentorship is often activated in a reactive way; for example, when something has gone wrong. Support should be about helping people learn rather than teaching them – getting people to stretch themselves and gain confidence to implement new ideas. By using opportunities in everyday situations to develop skills, increase knowledge and influence attitudes. The coaching role should be about training every person every day (Little, 2008). Success is based on what you do, not who you are. Behaviour can be learnt and unlearnt (Mann, 2005).

Conclusions

Effective leadership does not happen by chance or by the leader having the right personality. Effective clinical leadership is a skill where interpersonal communication is essential and leaders demonstrate passion and commitment to a vision of perfection. High quality of care for service users is also dependent on key staff continually striving to deliver a service that meets societal expectation. The organizational culture must foster teamworking and interdependent practices. Effective leadership must be evident at all levels and in all aspects of the whole organization.

Key points

- All staff have a role to play in shaping and leading service delivery.
- Leadership qualities should be continually developed and evaluated.
- Positive change cannot take place without emotional commitment.
- The organizational culture should foster openness and transparency.

Further reading

Balogun, J. and Hope Hailey, V. (2003) *Exploring Strategic Change*, 2nd edn. London: Prentice Hall.

Baird, A. (1998) Change theory and health promotion, *Nursing Standard*, 12(22): 34–6.

Bennett R, (1997) *Organizational Behavior*, 3rd edn. Essex: Pearson Education Ltd.

Burnes, B. (1996) *Managing Change: A Strategic Approach to Organizational Dynamics*, 2nd edn. London: Pitam.

Cameron, K.S., Quinn, R.E., Degraff, J. and Thakor, A.V. (2006) *Competing Values Leadership: Creating Value in Organizations*. Cheltenham: Edward Elgar Publishing Ltd.

Department of Health (DoH) (2004c) *Knowledge and Skills Framework*. London: DoH.

Feidler, F.A. (1967) *A Theory of Leadership Effectiveness*. New York: McGraw-Hill Education.

Frankl, V. (1963) *Man's Search for Meaning: An Introduction to Logotherapy*. New York: Washington Square Press.

Handy, C. (1999) *Understanding Organisations*, 4th edn. London: Penguin Books.

Iles, V. (1997) *Really Managing Health Care*. Maidenhead: Open University Press.

Johnson, G. and K. Scholes (1999) *Exploring Corporate Strategy*, 5th edn. London: Prentice Hall Europe.

Johnson, G. and Scholes, K. (1999) Cited in F. Graetz, M. Rimmer, A. Lawrence and A. Smith (2002) *Managing Organisational Change*. London: Wiley and Sons.

Locke, E.A. (1979) Cited in E.F. McKenna (2000) *Business Psychology and Organisational Behaviour: A Student's Handbook*. Hove: Psychology Press.

Skills for Care (2004) *Leadership and Management: A Strategy for Social Care Workforce*. Available online at www.skillsforcare.org.uk (accessed 7 February 2009).

Van Maurik, J. (2001) *Writers on Leadership*. London: Penguin Books.

Useful links

www.nursingleadership.co.uk (accessed 7 September 2009).

www.executive.modern.nhs.uk/ (accessed 28 October 2009).

www.NHSLeadershipQualities.nhs.uk (accessed 7 September 2009).

References

Adair, J. (1986) *Effective Team Building*. London: Pan.

Blanchard, K. and Hersey, P. (1977) *Management of Organisational Behaviour*, 3rd edn. Englewood Cliffs, NJ: Prentice Hall.

Buchanan, D. and Huczynski, A. (1997) *Organisational Behaviour: An Introductory Text*, 3rd edn. London: Prentice Hall.

Cameron, K.S. and Quinn, R.E. (2006) *Diagnosing and Changing Organizational Culture*. New York: John Wiley & Sons, Inc.

Covey, S. (1992) *The 7 Habits of Highly Effective People*. London: Simon & Schuster UK Ltd.

Covey, S.R. (2004) *The 8th Habit*. London: Simon & Schuster UK Ltd.

Denison, D., Hooijberg, R. and Quinn, R.E. (1995) Paradox and performance: toward a theory of behavioural complexity, *Managerial Leadership Organisational Science*, 6: 524–40.

Department of Health (DoH) (1999) *Making a Difference: Strengthening the Nursing, Midwifery and Health Visiting Contribution to Health and Healthcare*. London: DoH.

Department of Health (DoH) (2000a) *The NHS Plan: A Plan for Investment, a Plan for Reform*. London: DoH.

Department of Health (DoH) (2000b) *Meeting the Challenge: A Strategy for the Allied Health Professions*. London: DoH.

Department of Health (DoH) (2001) *The NHS Plan: An Action Guide for Nurses, Midwives and Health Visitors*. London: DoH.

Department of Health (DoH) (2002) *Managing For Excellence in the NHS*. London: DoH.

Department of Health (2004a) *The NHS Improvement Plan: Putting People at the Heart of Public Services*. London: DoH

Department of Health (DoH) (2004b) *National Standards, Local Action: Health and Social Care Standards and Planning Framework 2005/06–2007/08*. London: DoH.

Department of Health (DoH) (2004c) *Leadership and Management: A Strategy for the Social Care Workforce*. Leeds: Topss.

Department of Health (DoH) (2008) *Darzi Report High Quality Care for All: NHS Next Stage Review Final Report*. London: DoH

Gallo, C. (2007) *Fire Them Up! 7 Simple Secrets to: Inspire Colleagues, Customers and Clients; Sell Yourself, Your Vision, and Your Values; Communicate with Charisma and Confidence*. Danvers, MA: John Wiley and Sons, Inc.

Gladwell, M. (2000) *The Tipping Point: How Little Things can Make a Big Difference*. London: Abacus.

Goldsmith, M. and Reiter, M. (2007) *What Got You Here Won't Get You There, How Successful People Become Even More Successful*. New York: Hyperion.

Graetz, F., Rimmer, M., Lawrence, A., and Smith, A. (2002) *Managing Organisational Change*. Chichester: Wiley and Sons.

Grohar-Murray, M.E. and Dicroce, H.E. (2002) *Leadership and Management in Nursing*, 3rd edn. London: Pearson Education Ltd.

Hamilton, P.M. (1996) *Realities of Contemporary Nursing*, 2nd edn. Redwood, CA: Addison Wesley.

Hayes, J. (2002) *The Theory and Practice of Change Management*. Basingstoke: Palgrave Macmillan.

Kotter, J.P. (1996) *Leading Change*. Boston, MA: Harvard Business School Press.

Kouzes, J.M. and Posner, B.Z. (1995) *The Leadership Challenge*. San Fransisco, CA: Jossey-Bass.

Leigh, A. (2008) *The Charisma Effect: How to Make A Powerful and Lasting Impression*. London: Pearson Education/Prentice Hall.

Lewin, K. (1999) Cited in E.L.M Rigolosi (2005) *Management and Leadership in Nursing and Health Care: An Experiential Approach,* 2nd edn. New York: Springer Publishing Company.

Little, S. (2008) *The Milkshake Moment: Overcoming Stupid Systems, Pointless Policies and Muddled Management to Realize Real Growth.* Hoboken, NJ: John Wiley & Sons, Inc.

Locke, E.A. (1976) The nature and causes of job satisfaction, in M.D. Dunnette (ed.) *Handbook of Industrial and Organizational Psychology.* Chicago, IL: Rand McNally.

Mann, D. (2005) *Creating a Lean Culture: Tools to Sustain Lean Conversions.* New York: Productivity Press.

Marquis B.L. and Huston C.J. (1998) *Management Decision Making for Nurses: 124 Case Studies,* 3rd edn. Philadelphia, PA: Lippincott Williams & Wilkins.

McConnell, E. (1998) How to thrive in merger mania, *Journal of the Association of Perioperative Registered Nurses,* 67(2): 412–19.

Menix (2000) Cited in J. Daly, S. Speedy and D. Jackson (2004) *Nursing Leadership.* Australia: Elsevier.

Moss Kanter, R. (1989) *When Giants Learn to Dance: Mastering the Challenge of Strategy, Management, and Careers in the 1990s.* New York: Simon & Schuster, Inc.

NHS Institute for Innovation and Improvement (2005) *Improvement Leaders Guide: Leading Improvement, Personal and Organisational Development*: Coventry: NHS.

Perlman, D. and Takacs, G.J. (1990) The ten stages of change, *Nursing Management,* 21(4): 33.

Quinn, R. (2004) *Building the Bridge as you Walk on it: A Guide for Leading Change.* San Francisco, CA: Jossey-Bass.

Rogers, E. (1995) *The Diffusion of Innovations.* New York: The Free Press.

Seddon, J (2005) *Freedom from Command and Control: Rethinking Management for Lean Service.* New York: Productivity Press.

Shapiro A (2004) *Creating Contagious Commitment: Applying the Tipping Point to Organisational Change.* Hillsborough, NC: Strategy Perspective.

Sullivan, E.J. and Decker, P.J. (2009) *Effective Leadership and Management in Nursing,* 6th edn. Upper Saddle River, NJ: Pearson Education.

Wedderburn Tate, C. (1999) *Leadership in Nursing.* London: Churchill Livingstone.

3 | Whole systems approaches to organizational working

Rob McSherry

Introduction

This chapter briefly outlines why and how whole systems approaches to viewing and working in organizations can support the development of excellence in practice and oneself. It outlines what the terms and phrases mean and how this can be facilitated in practice. This is achieved by exploring origins and definitions of whole systems, providing evidence of whole systems in health and social care. It provides a practical example highlighting how whole systems approaches may support with the recurring issues of getting evidence into practice.

Background

The introduction of phrases, such as: systems thinking, systems reform, whole systems, systems theory, systems and processes and systems redesign are growing in popularity in health and social care (Stanton, 2007, cited in McSherry and Pearce, 2007). The incorporation, adoption and adaptation of systems approaches are primarily associated with improving the quality of the services and standards of care provided by individuals' teams and organization. The term 'systems theory' or 'whole systems approach' to which it is referred throughout this chapter is a relatively new approach in health and social care. However, it is important to highlight that it is not a new term or phrase to other disciplines or professions like business and engineering.

Basically, systems theory aims to provide an alternative approach to viewing problems and answering questions (von Bertalanffy, 1971). Systems theory according to von Bertalanffy (1974) was developed because modern classical sciences – physics, biology and chemistry – were failing to answer questions and solve problems, because of the reductionist, as opposed to the expansionist, approach to explaining social and biological phenomena. This is when the reduction goes from the broad to the specific, rather than focusing on the interactions and relationships between the sum and whole of the parts. For example, psychology is reduced to neurophysiology, neurophysiology to biochemistry and biochemistry to quantum physics. Skyttner (1996) argues that this kind of reductionism is both inefficient and ineffective in addressing complex problems. So where did the term 'whole systems approaches' emerge; what does it mean and what does it offer for health and social care organizations?

It would not be surprising to initially find Activity 3.1 challenging and difficult to undertake. This could be because you will not have heard of whole systems approaches or because you are familiar with the term and application guised in another way or a combination of both. The remainder of the chapter aims to offer you a step-by-step approach to raising your awareness of whole systems approaches.

⟳ Activity 3.1 Raising your awareness of whole systems approaches within health and social care

Whole systems approaches have undoubtedly become popular within health and social care organizations in resolving complex problems. Write down your answer to each of the following questions:

- Where does the term whole systems approaches originate?
- What do you understand by the term whole systems approaches?
- Why has the term whole systems approaches entered health and social care organizations?
- How may whole systems approaches support the workings of health and social care organizations?
- What are the potential advantages of using whole systems approaches to health and social care?
- Can you give any examples of where systems approaches have been used within health and social care?
- Can you highlight the types of whole systems approaches?

Read on and compare your notes with chapter content along with the activity feedback at the end of the chapter.

Where does the term 'whole systems approaches' originate from and what does it mean?

Ludwig von Bertalanffy, an Austrian biologist working in Vienna, introduced the term 'whole system' in the late 1920s when he wrote:

> since the fundamental character of the living thing is its organization, the customary investigation of the single parts and processes cannot provide a complete explanation of the vital phenomena. This investigation gives us no information about the coordination of parts and processes. Thus the

chief task of biology must be to discover the laws of biology systems (at all levels of organization) (von Bertalanffy, 1974: 410).

Von Bertalanffy called this type of investigation, 'organismic biology', but, in effect, he was explaining the system theory of the organism. Von Bertalanffy (1974) argued that organisms survive because of the complex interplay and relationships between the component parts that make up the whole organism.

Systems theory, offered by von Bertalanffy (1974), Boulding (1985), Rapoport (1986) and Skyttner (1996), provides an alternative to reductionism, through expansionism, which concentrates on understanding the function and behaviour of the whole system, as opposed to its separate parts. Systems approaches, according to Laszlo (1972), set out to understand and resolve complex situations by attempting to explain, not only their components, 'but also in regard to the entire set of relations between the components' (Laszlo, 1972: 5). Put simply, Skyttner (1996: 21) believes that systems theory, 'concentrates on the function and behaviour of the whole system'. Systems theorists, such as von Bertalanffy (1971, 1974), Laszlo (1972) and Skyttner (1996), support the ancient Aristotelian principles of the whole being more than the sum of its parts, which, during this period in history, had been demonized by the empirical sciences, because classical science was concerned with one-way causality, or relationships between two variables, as opposed to dealing with organized complexity.

Systems theory, according to Boulding (1985), is about establishing the interrelations between some, but not infinitely all, components of a problem. So why has whole systems approaches become popular in supporting health and social care organizations?

The emergence of whole systems approaches within health and social care

The popularity of systems theory has entered the health and social care arena, in the quest to resolve complex health and social care problems and in an attempt to improve the quality of care and services for patients (Rogers et al., 1999; Newhouse, 1999). Silbiger (1993) argues that whole systems approaches may be used to analyse the health status of an organization by reviewing the efficiency and effectiveness of the complex systems and processes that make up the 'whole' organization (Silbiger, 1993). Whole systems approaches are applicable to health and social care because: 'every healthcare operation, from an individual nursing unit to an entire healthcare system, has a structure, which is a key factor in system performance' (Keating and Morin, 2001: 357).

Based on the information provided above, it is easy to see why whole systems approaches have transcended into health and social care. This is because, as identified in Chapter 5, innovation and change, problem identification and resolution, quality, performance, outcome(s) and excellence are dependent

on how individuals and teams integrate and interact efficiently and effectively as part of the workings of the collective/combined organization.
Furthermore, quality and excellence are mutually dependent on how the
systems and processes they work with support the people or person in performing their role and executing the responsibilities both efficiently and
effectively. So how can whole systems approaches support the workings of a
health and social care organization?

Whole systems approaches supporting the workings of health and social care organizations

Whole systems approaches can support the workings of a health and social
care organization because, as highlighted in Chapter 1, it is about having
a vision and values that fosters shared working and shared governance.
That means having the openness, transparency and communications to
challenge and support the workings of the organizations in its pursuit of
excellence in practice. For example, for years health and social care professionals continue to struggle and grapple with the issue of getting evidence
into practice. Whole system approaches provide an opportunity to decipher
and understand the issues associated with getting evidence into practice,
for several reasons that we outline below.

Evidence-based practice

Scientists realized that the way they previously embraced and viewed the
world was not far-reaching enough to understand and explain what they
observed and encountered (Skyttner, 1996). The attempt to reduce complexities to their constituents and build an understanding of the wholeness,
through knowledge of its parts, is no longer valid. Classical health care, with
its overspecialization and compartmentalization has already proved its
inability to handle problems of increased complexity. For example, establishing the effects that the growing numbers of older people have on health and
social care systems cannot be achieved by focusing on just one aspect of the
problem. Similarly, it could be argued that it is not possible to decipher why
health care professionals struggle to get evidence into practice by focusing on
single issues, such as research awareness (Jolley, 2002) and decision-making
(Thompson, 1999). Adopting a whole systems approach, highlighted by von
Bertalanffy (1971, 1974), Laszlo (1972) and Skyttner (1996), seems applicable
in resolving the issues associated with getting evidence into practice. This is
because evidence-based practice is dependent, not only on identifying the
major elements deemed necessary for this to occur, like research awareness
and decision-making, but also on the following:

- having an appreciation of how the various elements and associated
  systems and processes connect

- how the various elements interact together as a whole
- how organizational cultures and working environments impact on these.

The notion of exploring complex organizational problems and solving problems, using an integrated manner, perhaps, explains why whole systems approaches have transcended to the psychosocial (Bowman, 1991); educational, via mathematical modelling and information theory (Klir, 1991); and health care (Checkland, 1981; Glasscock and Hales, 1998; Newhouse, 1999; Hronek and Bleich, 2002).

The purpose of whole systems approaches in all these instances is about solving problems and answering questions about complex situations. The emphasis is placed on improving the interconnectedness between the various systems and processes and showing how internal and external environmental factors affect the physical and non-physical infrastructures of the whole organization. Keating and Morin (2001) argue that the ultimate goal of whole systems theory is directed towards demonstrating performance in production and output of the organization. So what are the potential advantages of using whole systems approaches within health and social care?

Potential advantages of using whole systems approaches to health and social care

When transferring whole systems theory to the NHS and the problems associated with getting evidence into practice, some potential advantages emerge. Whole systems theory provides:

- a foundation for the structural analysis of the whole organization
- a way of accessing the health status of the organization and people working within and external to the organization
- a framework for assessing and measuring the effects of internal and external factors on the working environment
- a medium for analysing the efficiency and effectiveness of individuals, teams and departments on the whole, or aspects of the organization's performance and outcomes.

So what evidence is available to illustrate the relative merits and demerits of whole systems approaches within health and social care?

Example of whole systems approaches within health and social care

Some of the reported work on using whole systems approaches in the health and social care can be classified, broadly, into three areas: (1) organizational development and service improvement initiatives; (2) quality and performance; and (3) educational and professional developments.

Organizational development and service improvement initiatives

Systems theory, according to Rogers et al. (1999), Newhouse (1999) and Keating and Morin (2001), offers both a new and existing way of promoting and facilitating organizational development and service improvement within the NHS. Rogers et al. (1999) detail how improving access to NHS services and information during the winter, utilizing a whole systems approach, could avert a 'winter crisis' by informing the public and professionals about accessing services.

The organizational systems that were targeted centred on risk management, information and communication and performance management. The emphasis was placed on reviewing and evaluating past winter performances, and how existing systems and processes could be improved, to avoid future winter pressures; for example, bed blocking and closure to emergency admissions. The whole systems design took a 'people' approach, focusing on raising awareness about the need to access services during the winter months. The work targeted presenting the organization's access performance from the previous year(s) and the establishment of a multi-collaborative inter-agency approach to sharing and resolving the problem. 'Starting with the public involvement and working across the whole system, a coordinated strategy including joint working arrangements with social services, education, NHS ambulance trusts and pharmacists was put in place' (Rogers et al., 1999: 867).

The key output from the work was the development of a wider access strategy that enabled a pathway to be developed, implemented and evaluated, which focused specifically on how people access care during the winter.

Newhouse (1999), similarly to Rogers et al. (1999), reported on how whole systems theory can be used to offset, support or unite health and social care organizations, environments and cultures through turbulent times, such as mergers, consolidations and redesigns. Newhouse (1999) argues that whole systems should focus on the vertical approach to integration. Vertical integrated systems, unlike horizontal systems, which are created when the organization expands with similar products, services, or if several hospitals join together, provide health services and products to patients at multiple points along the lifespan. Vertical integrated systems have 'the capacity to provide, or arrange for the provision of, all types and levels of care required by its client population' (Nerenz and Zajac, 1996: 10). The strength of Newhouse's work to nurse executives, managers and administrators is in providing comprehensive guidance and support, with practical illustrations of how vertical integration systems could be the preferred method of developing, reviewing and evaluating health care provision in the future.

Keating and Morin (2001) illustrate the value of using a whole systems approach in determining and understanding operational and structural problems within an organization. The work provides useful theoretical foundations and models to support structural analysis of an organization. Keating and Morin (2001), by the utilization of a viable systems model

(VSM), highlight the significant system requirements for achieving a viable organization. These components should focus on ensuring that the organization's operations, coordination, controls, monitoring, development, learning and policy are continually improving. Furthermore, they provide practical guidance on how to structurally analyse the efficiency and effectiveness of these key components by the use of a four-phase analysis systems model. This model focuses on measuring and evaluating structure, process, outcomes and interpretations of the findings, a model not dissimilar in design to the quality frameworks forwarded by Donabedian (1966). The strength of a VSM approach to structural analysis is in providing nurse leaders, managers and executives with a framework that is easy to use and similar to previous quality measurement templates. Due to the familiarity and similarities of VSM, they could be applied and adopted to:

• enable deeper holistic evaluations of organizations systems and subsystems to be undertaken along with how the staff and public feel about the organization's performance
• diagnose structural faults and system failures of the organization's formal and informal frameworks in part or full; for example, the entire organization's performance for compliance with drugs policies or individual wards or departments.

The limitations of VSM are that they are time-consuming and require systematic planning, implementation and evaluation. On reviewing the works of Rogers et al. (1999), Newhouse (1999) and Keating and Morin (2001), it is easy to see the strength that whole systems theory has had in supporting structural reviews and developments within an organization. Systems theory in these cases is about improving efficiency and effectiveness of the whole system and its associated outcomes, or products. The weaknesses were in demonstrating the impact that key individuals (those who operate and perform within the systems and processes) have had on the overall performance and outcome of the whole system.

Quality and performance

The purpose of systems theory, according to Aikman et al. (1998), Page (1999), Hronek and Bleich (2002) and Hall (2002), is about improving the quality and performance of a service provided by an individual and/or organization. Aikman et al. (1998) argue that system integration is a necessity in enabling health care organizations to become more flexible, adaptive and responsive to innovation and change. The work details how a community teaching hospital transformed the way it provides services to its local community by building new systems and processes to service delivery. The strength of systems theory in this case was in encouraging partnership-building with local stakeholders by sharing responsibilities, fostering an open culture and a sound working relationship between staff and the public. The reported limitation of systems theory was the length of time and commitment required to embed the principles within the organization.

Similar to Aikman et al. (1998), Page (1999) highlights how systems theory enabled a strategy for performance improvement to be developed for a large acute 383-bed health care organization. The adoption of a whole systems approach facilitated the various departments and disciplines representing the provider network to be highlighted, along with the designated consumers, or defined population, linked to the service. As a consequence of this action, a shared vision and strategy was designed, having specific outcomes to meet the needs of both providers and consumers. Page (1999) argues that the long-term success of the performance improvement strategy will be dependent on four factors:

1 communication
2 leadership
3 decision-making *and*
4 effective team dynamics.

Unlike Page (1999) and Aikman et al. (1998), Hronek and Bleich (2002) utilized systems theory to review and improve the medication delivery system of a health care organization. Rather than focus on performance and outcome, Hronek and Bleich (2002) focused on reviewing and redesigning existing systems and processes for the recording, monitoring and evaluating of adverse medication events. The work showed that by focusing on adverse medication events, specific aspects of why medication systems and processes fail could be highlighted and resolved. These included recreating the infrastructure to support prescribing, procuring, dispensing and administration. Hall (2002), in contrast to Hronek and Bleich's (2002) emphasis on enhancing quality through reviewing and redesigning systems, arguing that systems do not make errors; people do. Hall (2002) provides several case scenarios where it was not the system at fault, but the people who operate them. Hall's alternative view of systems theory and quality suggests that fixing only the systems, without fixing the people who make errors, or do not want to engage with the systems and processes, will not work. Hall argues that errors made by staff may be prevented by changing the culture and practice of believing that errors are made by systems instead of by people.

Educational and professional development

The education and professional development of staff play a major role in creating a quality organization and effective clinical environment. Wells's (1995) study aimed to improve how in-patient psychiatric nurses, working on an acute mental health admissions unit, are prepared for innovation and change. Wells (1995) applied Checkland's (1981) 'soft systems methodology' (SSM) to review educational activity on the ward by observing practice and reviewing documentation over a two-month period. From this data a rich picture of reality was drawn, and a conceptual model developed, highlighting the key differences between actuality and those activities required to change and enhance practice. The study showed that in order to improve the discharge planning process, staff require support from the local educational college in devising a discharge development programme and ongoing education and training for staff.

Since Wells's (1995) study was reported, several larger studies have utilized SSM to highlight the impact of practice development (Clarke and Wilcockson, 2001) and education initiatives (Clarke and Wilcockson, 2001; Stokes and Lewin, 2004) on individual and organizational practice. Clarke and Wilcockson's (2001, 2002) studies identify the strengths, weaknesses, opportunities and threats of using soft systems approaches for those uninitiated in systems theory. Furthermore, they highlighted how SSM can be applied to review professional and organizational learning and the challenges of using evidence in nursing practice. Stokes and Lewin (2004), unlike Clarke and Wilcockson (2001, 2002), demonstrate the usefulness of SSM in highlighting the information-seeking behaviour of a group of lecturers, delivering a nursing and midwifery programme. The small-scale study highlighted a diverse range of information-seeking behaviours, covering peer-reviewed journals and accessing libraries. More significant was the fact that systems theory allowed the analysis of a broad and complex situation to be reviewed, which enabled changes to information-seeking behaviours of lecturers to be implemented.

In contrast to the formal studies of Wells (1995), Stokes and Lewin (2004) and Clarke and Wilcockson (2001, 2002), Glasscock and Hales (1998) demonstrate how they used systems theory to introduce Bowmen's (1991) principles of what constitutes a functional family unit, to nursing management, to explain why problems experienced by individual team members affect the function of an entire group. The incorporation of Bowmen's (1991) framework meant that problems, such as conflict, absenteeism, productivity slowdowns, low morale and individual inadequacies, could be viewed as system problems, rather than as an individual problem. Any member of an organization, group, or team, therefore, can affect and influence change in the system.

Types of whole systems approach

System theorists, Checkland (1981) and Skyttner (1996), suggest that systems can be classified into two types; hard (Skyttner, 1996) and soft (Checkland, 1981).

Hard systems

Skyttner (1996) argues that hard system methodologies involve using concepts as a means of investigating complex situations, and taking rational action, with the objective of achieving what are seen to be defined, unquestioned and, frequently, unproblematic goals. Hard systems, according to Skyttner (1996), work because of the implicit belief that any problem can be solved by setting objectives and finding optimal satisfying alternatives, directed towards a defined problem solution. Identifying, designing and implementing are the main phases of this approach, which is why they are used, generally, in the field of systems engineering and systems analysis, where a specific piece of equipment requires developing, or adaptation to an existing electrical system, due to the development of a fault that requires correcting.

Soft systems

Soft systems, in contrast to hard systems, according to Checkland and Scholes (1990: 1) 'is an organised way of tackling messy situations in the real world. It is based on systems thinking, which enables it to be highly defined and described, but is flexible in use and broad in scope'. Checkland (1981) argues that underpinning the soft system method is the belief that in a problem situation there is often a sense of discontent without focus: 'characterised by a sense of mismatch, which eludes precise definition, between what is perceived to be actually and what is perceived might become reality' (Checkland, 1981: 5).

The adoption or adaptation of whole systems approaches within any working organization advocates an interdisciplinary and holistic approach by bringing together fragmentary research findings in a comprehensive view of people, nature and society. Perhaps this is why a whole systems approach or theory is defined as:

> a logical mathematical field whose task is the formulation and derivation of those general principles that are applicable to 'systems' in general. In this way exact formulations of terms such as wholeness and sum, differentiation, progressive mechanization, centralization, hierarchical order, finality and equinfinality, etc ... become possible, terms which occur in all sciences dealing with 'systems' and imply their logical homology (von Bertalanffy, 1974: 411).

By taking Skyttner's (1996) and Checkland's (1981) four points into account, a system could be regarded as an entity, which can maintain some organization in the face of change, from within, or without. To review a system efficiently and effectively, however, requires the utilization of a robust system theory methodology using either or both hard and soft system approaches.

The above review demonstrates the enormous potential that systems theory holds in problem identification and solution, when a complex organizational system and process, such has those aligned to health and social care, is faced with change. If introduced and managed effectively, systems theory has the potential to support organizational and service improvement and the performance and quality agendas by targeting specific, or whole parts, of the system; for instance, reviewing why health and social care professionals are not using evidence in support of their practice, or why there are rising numbers of reported clinical incidents. Despite the positive contribution in problem recognition and solving, however, the success of systems theory is dependent on identifying and applying an appropriate systems theory and methodology. It is imperative, therefore, to establish what the principles of systems theory are and to see if they can be modified and applied to this context.

Case study 3.1 Applying whole systems approaches to support getting evidence into practice

Despite the upsurge in evidence over the past decade, registered nurses continue to struggle to get evidence into practice.

The following case study illustrates how the application of a whole systems approach has enabled the development of the evidence-informed nursing (EIN) model designed with the intention of facilitating evidence into practice.

Source: Adapted from McSherry (2006)

Why was the EIN model developed?

In brief the EIN model was developed to offer nurses (indeed all health and social care professionals) a systematic approach to providing evidence-based nursing care, which requires individual nurses to have:

- an understanding of the importance of practice being based on the most appropriate evidence on effectiveness;
- access to and ability to use research findings;
- the ability to evaluate research and the ability to implement research findings in their own practice.

How did a whole systems approach enable the EIN model to be developed?

According to Skyttner (1996) and Checkland (1981) whole systems approaches should include: defining a system; formulating a taxonomy of systems; singling out properties that various systems have in common; and explaining how this approach can help us to have a better understanding of the world. Put simply, Skyttner (1996) and Checkland (1981) purport the following stages in developing a system.

Stage 1 Identifying and outlining the system

The EIN model was designed following a critical review of the various evidence-based definitions and models and frameworks by drawing together a selection of elements and their associated systems and processes deemed necessary to denote how nurses inform their nursing practice with evidence.

Stage 2 What constitutes the components/parts to the system?

Skyttner (1996) argues that a system can be categorized into four general categories: concrete; conceptual; abstract; and unperceivable, each having basic, operational, purposive, or controlling functions as identified in Table 3.1.

Based on Table 3.1, the EIN model could be regarded as having an operational and purposive function, because it aims to encourage registered nurses to apply and evaluate the effectiveness of using evidence in practice through the operation of a series of single elements within a whole system. The EIN model could be classified as a conceptual system due to the fact that it consists of a series of elements that when unified provide a basis for getting evidence into practice. The elements are professional accountability, informed decision-making, research awareness, application of knowledge, evaluation and conditions affecting nursing research utilization. Furthermore, Skyttner (1996) argues that it is important to explain that systems can be 'open'; dependent on the environment with which to exchange matter, energy and information, and/or, 'closed'; open for input of energy only. Both

Table 3.1 Types of system

System category	Description	Example of system type
Concrete	Exists in the physical reality of space and time and is defined as living and non-living	Human species
Conceptual	Composed of an organization of ideas expressed in symbolic form. Its units may be words, numbers or other symbols. A conceptual system can only exist in some form of concrete system	A newly devised database for intermediate care housed and run by a computer
Abstract	All elements are concepts	An organizational chart
Unperceivable	As many parts and complicated interrelationships between them hiding the actual structure of the system	The universe

open and closed systems, however, may be influenced by space (environment); for example, the complexities of a nurse getting evidence into practice is dependent on the unification of a series of complex open systems and sub-systems associated with informed decision-making (Thompson, 1999), which can be promoted, or hindered, by the organization's culture and working environment (Kitson et al., 1998).

Stage 3 Putting the system together

Rapoport (1986) argues that for a system to exist requires four other common elements to work efficiently and effectively: *input, throughput* (process), *output* and *feedback* (evaluation). The critical review of existing models and frameworks and evidence-based definitions indicate that Rapoport's (1996) system requirements of the EIN model could be summarized in Figure 3.1.

Figure 3.1 shows that the working elements of the EIN model are inextricably linked to the eight elements associated with getting evidence into practice. The *input* to the system is informed by the fact that registered nurses

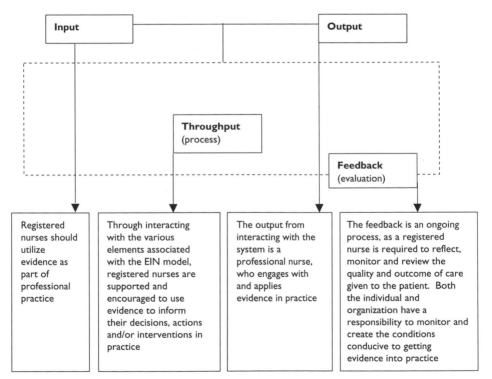

Input	Output

Throughput (process)

Feedback (evaluation)

| Registered nurses should utilize evidence as part of professional practice | Through interacting with the various elements associated with the EIN model, registered nurses are supported and encouraged to use evidence to inform their decisions, actions and/or interventions in practice | The output from interacting with the system is a professional nurse, who engages with and applies evidence in practice | The feedback is an ongoing process, as a registered nurse is required to reflect, monitor and review the quality and outcome of care given to the patient. Both the individual and organization have a responsibility to monitor and create the conditions conducive to getting evidence into practice |

Figure 3.1 Summarizing the working elements of the EIN model

are required by the NMC, employer and public to practise using best evidence.

Both registered nurses and employing organizations have a role and responsibility in ensuring that this happens. The *process* of registered nurses using evidence in practice is dependent on them becoming informed of what the elements are and how they promote evidence-based nursing. Likewise, the employing organization needs to put in place a series of processes that empower and encourage the utilization of evidence into practice; for example, raising awareness of the various elements of evidence-based nursing and developing an organizational culture and context that are conducive to getting evidence into practice. Equally, registered nurses and NHS organizations have a shared responsibility to monitor and evaluate the impact of their decision and/or action in and on practice. If the system is working efficiently and effectively, the *output* is a professional nurse, an organizational culture and working environment that promote and practice evidence-based nursing. The challenge is in showing how the elements that make up the whole system and sub-systems interconnect, as well as the flow of communication between the various parts, so that the problem under review can be studied as a whole.

When compared to the works of systems theorists, like Ackoff (1981) and Pratt et al. (1999), the pooled evidence from the previous sections indicates that the theoretical EIN model (Figure 3.1) provides an integrated framework for registered nurses and organizations to use, to get evidence into practice. The importance of this framework is that it is based on informing the person(s) about the rationale behind evidence-based nursing, the processes involved and how this may be achieved by engaging with the key elements.

The *person*, as highlighted previously, is associated with ensuring that individual registered nurses and their employing organizations understand the drivers for, and origins of evidence-based nursing, the relative merits and demerits of engaging with the processes and how this is dependent on the nature of the individual, the culture and context of the organization. Practising evidence-based nursing requires enthusiasm and a willingness to accept and respond to change. Registered nurses need to be informed of the fact that evidence-based nursing is a complex and multidimensional process. To practise evidence-based nursing, they require new knowledge, understanding, skills and confidence associated with what constitutes evidence. Furthermore, they require a level of research awareness to resolve the conditions that support or hinder them from applying evidence in support of their practice.

The *process*, according to systems theorists (von Bertalanffy, 1974; Miller, 1978; Boulding, 1985; Rapoport, 1986), involves a series of changes by which something or someone develops as a consequence of going through a series, or number of steps. To achieve evidence-based nursing, an individual needs

to have the research awareness skills, knowledge and competence to interpret research material to inform their clinical decision-making, along with a
managerial and organizational culture that aids the implementation of
research (Cullum et al., 1998). Furthermore, Kitson et al. (1998), McCormack
et al. (1999) and Rycroft-Malone et al. (2004) argue that evidence-based
nursing requires facilitation. Facilitation, in this instance, is about informing
nurses of the 'processes' associated with the eight elements that constitute
the EIN model. Figure 3.1 illustrates how the EIN model is dynamic and
multidimensional in the way it uses modified whole system theory (MWST)
as a means of integrating the numerous elements that collectively constitute
evidence-based nursing. The EIN model would appear almost linear in nature,
yet the reality of this occurring in practice is much more messy, complex and
challenging.

For evidence-based nursing to occur, it requires the processing and communication of information between and within the various *elements* of the
system. For registered nurses to engage with the evidence, they need to be
aware of the drivers for getting evidence into practice (E1) and that using
evidence is an integral part of their professional role and responsibility (E2).
To utilize evidence in practice, the registered nurse, as part of their decision-
making process, should be able to use a problem-solving approach (E4) to
assess and prioritize the individual needs of the patient. Furthermore, by
having a knowledge of evidence-based nursing (E3) and sound research
awareness skills, the registered nurse should be able to access and critically
appraise the various forms of evidence (E5) to inform their practice. Registered nurses should be able to appreciate the challenges of getting evidence
into practice, and how these may be resolved (E6). Finally, the registered
nurse should devise individual strategies and engage with organizational
strategies to evaluate the efficiency and effectiveness of their decision, action
or intervention in practice (E7). By engaging successfully, in elements
(E1–E7), hopefully, it will result in a professional nurse (E8); someone who
is happy to challenge, question, and base practice on best evidence. Put
simply, the input (I) evidence supported by developing the elements (E1–E7)
results with an output (O) of improved quality care and a professional
nurse (E8).

Stage 4 Outcome or benefit from developing the system

The failure of a registered nurse and/or organization to become informed
about what these elements entail and how these can be developed could
result in poor standards of nursing care, undesired patient outcomes, along
with an organizational culture and working environment that is not conducive to getting evidence into practice. Whole systems approaches show
how the theoretical EIN model can be framed in supporting registered nurses
to become sufficiently informed in order to practice using an evidence base.

Attribution of whole systems approaches to nursing

According to Bertalanffy (1971, 1974), Boulding (1985), Rapoport (1986) and Skyttner (1996), a system requires definitions in terms of the formulation of the elements that constitute the system, the singling out of properties that the various systems have in common and an explanation of how this approach can help us to understand the problem under review. The EIN model (Figure 3.1), when compared and contrasted to the work of system theorists, von Bertalanffy (1971, 1974), Rapoport (1986) and Skyttner 1996), seems to have the potential characteristics and attributes deemed necessary to be regarded as a system. This is because the EIN model can be shown to meet the system theory criteria as follows.

The EIN model can be shown to demonstrate compliance and adherence to systems theory criteria for the following reasons:

- The EIN model has been *defined* and conceptualized from the pooled evidence gathered from the critical review of the evidence-based definitions and existing models and frameworks.
- The EIN model has a specific *goal* of encouraging and enabling registered nurses to use evidence in practice.
- The EIN model is an *open dynamic system*. This is because its success is dependent on the interconnectedness and communication between the various elements that constitute the model, along with the development of sound relationships between the individual registered nurse and the organizational culture and context of their working environment.
- The EIN model has a well-defined *input*, the use of 'evidence', *throughput*, associated with empowering registered nurses to engage with the eight elements, and an anticipated *output*, of improving decision-making and professional practice. The system's *boundaries* outline the importance of having clearly defined lines of accountability.
- Accountability within the EIN model can be directed at three levels: *individual, organizational* and *shared*. *Individually* – registered nurses are reminded of the need to use evidence to support their decisions and action as part of their code of professional practice and contract of employment. *Organizationally* – the employer is reminded of the major role they have in supporting and facilitating registered nurses to use evidence in practice. Both the individual and organization, however, need to be made aware of the *shared* responsibility they have of informing each other about any issues that they feel hinder the use of evidence in practice. Whether positive or negative, the consequences of registered nurses and organizations engaging with the EIN model are highlighted under the criterion – *entropy*. Entropy, according to Skyttner (1996), is associated with the degree of disorder in a system. In this instance, entropy pertains to establishing the degree of engagement with the evidence, and what conditions promote or hinder this from happening at an individual and/or organizational level.

- Finally, systems associated with controlling, monitoring and evaluating the EIN model to highlight achievement of, or divergence from its goal, can be shown to exist under the guise of *control* and *equifinality*.

The future of whole systems reform to health and social care organizations and working

Systems theory, offered by von Bertalanffy (1974), Boulding (1985), Rapoport (1986) and Skyttner (1996), provides an alternative to reductionism, through expansionism, which concentrates on understanding the function and behaviour of the whole system, as opposed to its separate parts. Systems approaches, according to Laszlo (1972), set out to understand and resolve complex situations by attempting to explain, not only their components, 'but also in regard to the entire set of relations between the components' (Laszlo, 1972: 5). Put simply, Skyttner (1996: 21) believes that systems theory, 'concentrates on the function and behaviour of the whole system'. Scientists realized that the way they previously embraced and viewed the world was not far-reaching enough to understand and explain what they observed and encountered (Skyttner, 1996). The attempt to reduce complexities to their constituents and build an understanding of the wholeness, through knowledge of its parts, is no longer valid. Classical health care with its overspecialization and compartmentalization has already proved its inability to handle problems of increased complexity.

Conclusion

Whole systems approaches offer a fantastic opportunity for enhancing the workings of an organization in the quest for quality and excellence. This is because whole systems approaches focus on problem identification and solution when a complex organizational system and process, such as those aligned to health and social care, is faced with challenge and change. Whole systems approaches can also highlight areas for celebration and offer acknowledgement of dedication, commitment by highlighting where and why things are working well. If introduced and managed effectively, whole systems approaches have the potential to support organizational and service improvement and the performance and quality agendas by targeting specific, or whole parts, of the system. Despite the positive contribution in problem recognition and solving, the success of whole systems approaches is dependent on identifying and applying an appropriate systems theory and methodology. It is imperative, therefore, to establish what the principles of systems theory are and to see if they can be modified and applied to this context.

↻ **Activity 3.2 Feedback**

The term 'whole systems' is a highly complex and technical term to decipher and operationalize on a daily basis. Whole systems approaches offer new and creative ways of promoting excellence in practice through taking a holistic or integrated approach to developing, redesigning or evaluating the workings of an organisation. Whole systems approaches are proven to offer new ways of working and in enhancing quality and services by encouraging people to embrace innovation and change at an individual, team and organizational level. Furthermore, whole systems approaches focus on the input, throughput and outputs of quality services.

Key points

- Whole system approaches aim to provide an alternative approach to viewing problems and answering questions.
- The popularity of systems theory has entered the health and social care arena, in the quest to resolve complex health and social care problems, in an attempt to improve the quality of care and services for patients.
- Systems theory provides an alternative to reductionism through expansionism, which concentrates on understanding the function and behaviour of the whole system, as opposed to its separate parts.
- Innovation and change, problem identification and resolution, quality, performance, outcome(s) and excellence are dependent on how individuals and teams integrate and interact efficiently and effectively as part of the workings of the collective/combined organization.
- The ultimate goal of whole systems theory is directed towards demonstrating performance in production and output of the organization.
- Whole systems approaches in health and social care can be classified broadly into three areas: organizational development and service improvement initiatives; quality and performance; and educational and professional developments.
- Systems can be classified into two types: hard and soft.
- Whole systems approaches offer a fantastic opportunity for enhancing the workings of an organization in the quest for quality and excellence.

Useful links

Davis, G. (2005) *Soft Systems Methodology*. Canada: University of Calgary. Available online at www.guydavis.ca/seng/seng613/summaries/ssm.shtml (accessed 7 July 2009).

References

Ackoff, R. (1981) *Creating the Corporate Future*. New York: John Wiley and Sons, Inc.

Aikman, P., Andress, I., Goodfellow, C., LaBelle, N. and Porter-O'Grady, T. (1998) System integration: a necessity, *Journal of Nursing Administration*, 28(2): 28–34.

Bertalanffy, L. von (1971) *General System Theory: Foundations, Development and Applications*. London: Allen Lane/The Penguin Press.

Bertalanffy, L. von (1974) The history and status of general systems theory, *Academy of Management Journal*, 15(4): 407–26.

Bowmen, M. (1991) Alcoholism as viewed through family systems theory and family psychotherapy, *Family Dynamic Addict Q*, 1(1): 94–102.

Boulding, K. (1985) *The World as a Total System*. London: Sage Publications.

Bowmen, M. (1991) Alcoholism as viewed through family systems theory and family psychotherapy, *Family Dynamic Addict Q*, 1(1): 94–102.

Checkland, P. (1981) *Systems Thinking, Systems Practice*. Chichester: Wiley and Sons:

Checkland, P. and Scholes, J. (1990) *Soft Systems Methodology in Action*. Chichester: Wiley and Sons.:

Clarke, C.L. and Wilcockson, J. (2001) Professional and organizational learning: analysing the relationship with the development of practice, *Journal of Advanced Nursing*, 34(2): 264–72.

Clarke, C.L. and Wilcockson, J. (2002) Seeing need and developing care: exploring knowledge for and from practice, *International Journal of Nursing Studies*, 39(4): 397–406.

Cullum, N., DiCenso, A. and Ciliska, D. (1998) Implementing evidence-based nursing: some misconceptions, *Evidence-based Nursing*, 1(2): 38–40.

Donabedian, A. (1966) Evaluating the quality of medical care MIL, *MEM.FUND.QU* XLIV, 3(2): 166–203.

Glasscock, F.E. and Hales, A. (1998) Bowen's family systesms theory: a useful approach for a nurse administrator's practice, *Journal of Nursing Administrator*, 28(6): 37–42.

Hall, J.K. (2002) Systems don't make mistakes – people do, *JONAS Healthcare Law Ethics Regulation*, 4(2): 1–5.

Hronek, C. and Bleich, M.R. (2002) The less-than-perfect medication system: a systems approach to improvement, *Journal of Nursing Care Quality*, 16(4): 17–22.

Jolley, S. (2002) Raising research awareness: a strategy for nurses, *Nursing Standard*, 16(33): 33–9.

Keating, C. and Morin, M. (2001) An approach for systems analysis of patient care operations, *Journal of Nursing Administration*, 31(7/8): 355–63.

Kitson, A.L., Harvey, G. and McCormack, B. (1998) Enabling the implementation of evidence based practice: a conceptual model, *Quality Health Care*, 7: 149–58.

Laszlo, E. (1972) *The Relevance of General Systems Theory*. New York: George Braziller, Inc.

McCormack, B., Manley, K., Kitson, A., Titchen, A. and Harvey, G. (1999) Towards practice development: a vision in reality or reality without vision, *Journal of Nursing Management*, 7(5): 255–64.

McSherry, R. (2006) Developing, exploring and refining a modified whole systems based model of evidence-informed nursing. Unpublished PhD thesis, University of Teesside, Middlesbrough, England.

McSherry, R. and Pearce, P. (2007) *Clinical Governance: A Guide to Implementation for Healthcare Professionals*, 2nd edn. Oxford: Blackwell.

Miller, J. (1978) *Living Systems*. New York: McGraw-Hill.

Nerenz, D.R. and Zajac, B.M. (1996) Assessing performance of integrated delivery systems: analyzing indicators and reporting results, in Faulkner and Gray's *Medical Outcomes and Practice Guidelines Library*, volume 5. New York: Faulkner and Gray.

Newhouse, R.P. (1999) Vertical systems integration, *Journal of Nursing Administration*, 29(10): 22–9.

Page, C.K. (1999) Performance improvement integration: a whole systems approach, *Journal of Nursing Care Quality*, 13(3): 59–70.

Pratt, J., Gordon, P. and Plamping, D. (1999) *Working Whole Systems: Putting Theory into Practice in Organisations*. London: King's Fund.

Rapoport, A. (1986) *General System Theory: Essential Concepts and Applications*. Cambridge: Abacus Press.

Rogers, A., Flowers, J. and Pencheon, D. (1999) Improving access needs a whole systems approach: and will be important in averting crises in the millennium winter, *British Medical Journal*, 319(7214): 866–7.

Rycroft-Malone, J., Seers, K., Titchen, A., Harvey, G.B., Kitson, A. and McCormack, B. (2004) What counts as evidence in evidence-based practice? *Journal of Advance Nursing*, 47(10): 81–90.

Silbiger, S. (1993) *The 10 Day MBA*. London: Butler and Tanner Ltd.

Skyttner, L. (1996) *General Systems Theory: An Introduction*. London: Macmillan Press Ltd.

Stokes, P.JK. and Lewin, D. (2004) Information-seeking behaviour of nurse teachers in a school of health studies: a soft systems analysis, *Nurse Education Today*, 24(1): 47–54.

Thompson, C. (1999) A conceptual treadmill: the need for 'middle ground' in clinical decision making theory in nursing, *Journal of Advanced Nursing*, 30(5): 1222–9.

Wells, J.S.G. (1995) Discontent without focus? An analysis of nurse management and activity on a psychiatric in-patient facility using a 'soft systems' approach, *Journal of Advanced Nursing*, 21(2): 214–21.

PART 2
Collaborative working

4 | Cross-professional working and development

Sarah Hean

Introduction

Changes in service organization in health and social care have led to increased requirements for teamworking between different health and social care professionals and, often simultaneously, to a blurring and overlapping of traditional professional role boundaries. The public inquiries into the deaths of children undergoing cardiac surgery at the Bristol Royal Infirmary (Department of Health (DoH), 2001) and the death of Victoria Climbie (DoH, 2003) have demonstrated that these cross-professional teams do not always work optimally, leading to a lack of continuity of, (Service Delivery Organization (NHS/SDO), 2001), or even serious errors, in care. It is therefore essential that practitioners involved in practice development have an understanding of the dimensions and challenges to cross-professional teamworking.

A clear articulation of some of the principles underpinning cross-professional teamworking is important for practitioners as these principles provide practical tools to enable team members and managers to reflect, articulate, identify dilemmas and improve practice. It can assist with predictions and plans for working with and between health and social care colleagues. If practitioners are not conscious of the theoretical underpinnings of their actions, it could be argued that this brings their professional accountability into question. Such awareness is particularly important when practitioners face times of change (as practitioners do in the current health and social care system – Eraut, 2003). This chapter presents some tools with which practitioners may use and apply to articulate their cross professional practice.

Defining cross-professional working

A first step in this direction is to develop an understanding of the variation in the type of teams that exist and the terminology used to describe how different professional groups come together when working within them. Although clear distinctions are drawn between terms, these are still used interchangeably and with some confusion (Hall and Weaver, 2001; Miller et al., 2001; Thylefors et al., 2005).

Uni-professional teamworking

Uni-professional teamworking occurs within teams comprising of only one professional group. Challenges and structures that apply to all forms of team and collaborative working discussed elsewhere in this book will apply. The team tasks do not involve collaboration across professional boundaries.

Cross-professional teamworking

Thylefors et al. (2005) recommend the generic use of the term 'cross-professional' to encompass all teams in which several professional groups are represented. These include teams that exhibit either multi or inter-professional working. These two forms of cross-professional working can be distinguished by the specialization of the role of each professional, the inter-dependence of the task they perform, the coordination that is required to achieve this task, the specialization of the task involved and the interdependence of the roles within the team (Thylefors et al., 2005). In multi-professional teams a range of professionals share a common goal; for example, treatment of the patient but little interaction or coordination of activities occurs between professional groups involved in the care pathway. Working in parallel and duplication of effort is common. Inter-professional teamworking, however, is achieved in a more interactive and cooperative manner, where active coordination of activities takes place. A more detailed discussion of the above and other relevant terminology and its uses can be reviewed in discussion by (Hall and Weaver, 2001; Miller et al., 2001; Thylefors et al., 2005).

Cross-professional teams are not necessarily only made up of health and social care professionals. Police, lawyers, teachers, probation officers, and so on are also part of the wider cross-professional team involved in the care of the client's needs.

⟳ **Activity 4.1**

Think of your own practice and identify and describe the aspects of your work that represent:

- uni-professional teamworking
- multi-professional teamworking
- inter-professional teamworking.

- List the professionals involved in the team.
- List the activities in which each professional group is involved.
- Describe the overlap between these activities.
- Describe how this overlap is managed or coordinated by the team.

Read on and compare your answers with the rest of the chapter.

The outcomes of an effective cross-professional team

As delivery and organization of health and social care becomes increasingly dependent on team functioning, it is reassuring that evidence suggests that teamworking does improve patient care. Borrill et al. (2001) investigated a sample of community health care teams, primary health care teams and secondary health care teams. They concluded that there is a significant and negative relationship between the percentage of staff working in teams and patient mortality. In other words, the more people who are members of a team in an organization, the better the outcomes for the patient.

However, no single outcome can define whether a team is effective or not. Patient mortality is not the only outcome measure of an effective team and in some cases may be inappropriate (e.g. in a palliative care team where the patient's quality of life and well-being are more appropriate measures of effectiveness). Patient-focused outcomes are central but measurements of staff-related factors, such as improved staff mental health, are also valid team outcomes (Borrill et al., 2001).

There is surprisingly only limited research comparing the effectiveness of the cross-professional teams over uni-professional ones and the effectiveness of the inter-professional team over the less integrated multi-professional teams. Thylefors et al. (2005) reviewed some of this evidence and showed further that the greater the level of integration within the cross-professional team, the more likely were these teams to be rated highly in terms of perceived efficiency and team climate. A list of other positive outcomes from a cross-professional team is presented in Table 4.1.

Table 4.1 Some outcomes of an effective cross-professional team

Direct benefits to patient (Miller et al., *2001)*	*Benefits to team-indirect benefits (Borrill and West, 2000; Borrill et al., 2001; Thylefors et al., 2005)*
• *Continuity of care* (e.g. being able to carry over care when the experts are absent) • *Reduction of ambiguity:* no conflicting messages being given to patients • *Appropriate and timely referral:* each member has knowledge of another's professional roles and also their boundaries and hence able to judge accurately when it is appropriate to refer a patient to another member of their team • *Action and decisions based in a holistic perspective:* discussion between members leads to a holistic view of the patient • *Actions and decisions based on problem solving:* discussion and dissemination of knowledge between members is possible	• *Decreased team member turnover* • *Good mental health within team members* • *Good team climate* • *Cost-effectiveness* • *High self and external ratings of general team effectiveness* • *High self and external ratings of the quality of health care delivered by the team* • *High self and external ratings of innovation within the team's practice*

Ↄ **Activity 4.2 Cross-professional teamworking**

Think of the cross-professional team within which you work and consider the following:

- Identify three patient-related outcomes of the team and three staff related outcomes.
- How might you measure/evaluate the level of these outcomes?
- Would these outcomes be possible within a uni-professional team?
- Which of these are only possible through cross-professional teamworking?

Read on and compare your answers with the rest of the chapter

How positive outcomes are achieved within a cross-professional team

How do we as practitioners develop cross-professional teams that can achieve the positive outcomes outlined in Table 4.1? Unfortunately, this will not be a straightforward list of 'do's and don'ts' as there will never be a definitive list of the ideal team composition or optimum processes that will make any individual team effective. This is because the concept of effectiveness has many dimensions. A team may be effective on one of these but not another. Therefore, the characteristics of a team that may be good at achieving one particular outcome may not be suitable if different outcomes are focused on. For example, Borrill et al. (2001) measured the effectiveness of a cross-professional team through assessing levels of innovation shown by the team. In this instance, it is understandable that large teams with a diverse range of professions, each contributing a wealth of diverse ideas, would be better able to support and achieve this outcome. If the outcome measures had related to other outcomes, such as staff cohesion and mental health, the findings may have been very different where a smaller, more homogeneous team may have been perceived as more successful.

Despite the fact that the type of team may have different optimum requirements, based on its own nature as well as the outcome measure used, there are common attributes of a good cross-professional team that arise. A useful classification of these may be achieved by superimposing the concept of social capital onto these conditions.

Social capital is a heuristic concept used to describe, understand and measure the advantages gained by individual(s) who are part of a social network (Hean et al., 2002). The social network of interest here is the cross-professional team. The advantages of team membership are viewed in Table 4.1. The components of the team that need to be in place to achieve these benefits can be classified by main components of social capital (Hean et al., 2002), which are:

- the physical characteristics of the network (e.g. frequency of participation in network, size, homogeneity)
- the norms and rules that govern processes within it
- the external resources available to it (resources outside of the individual team member; e.g. financial resources)
- internal resources (resources within each team member; e.g. self-efficacy)
- trust in other team members.

A range of factors that fall under each of the above dimensions can be viewed in Table 4.2.

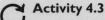 **Activity 4.3**

From your answer to Activity 4.2 identify a desired outcome of your cross-professional team.

- Describe your cross-professional team in terms of the components of social capital outlined in Table 4.1.
- How might each of these components be improved to achieve the desired outcome of your team?

Read on and compare your answers with the rest of the chapter.

Different philosophies and stereotyping: challenges to inter-professional working

Despite best intentions, there are a variety of reasons that cross-professional teams do not function optimally and the social capital potential of these teams is not achieved. The first relates to the *norms and rules* component of the network/team: the importance of a shared philosophy of working within the cross-professional team. The second is the presence of inter-professional stereotypes that may limit the *internal resources* of cross-professional flexibility, articulation and appreciation.

Philosophies

Miller et al. (2001) identified through observations of cross-professional teams three different team philosophies of working within them: a directive philosophy, an integrative philosophy and an elective philosophy. A

Table 4.2 Examples of some components of social capital to consider when developing the multi-professional team

Network characteristics	Norms and rules	External resources	Internal resources	Trust
• Frequency and nature of participation in team • Heterogeneity/homogeneity of group in terms of professional group • Longevity and stability of team • Staff tenure (part time/full time) • Size of team • Geographical location of team members	• Commitment to quality • Clarity of objectives • Clarity of leadership/coordination • Shared values or philosophies of working	• Physical mechanisms to support goals of team • Peer support • Strategies for conflict resolution • Financial resources	• Appreciation of how other disciplines understand knowledge and the methods by which it is gained and used • Flexibility that includes valuing different perspectives, accepting changes and a willingness to take on challenges • Reflexivity • Disciplinary articulation: all members understanding each other's role and recognizing areas of overlap within the traditional disciplinary boundaries	• Team climate

Source: (Borrill and West, 2000; Borrill et al., 2001; Miller et al. 2001; Thylefors et al., 2005)

directive philosophy was frequently held by members of the medical profession and non-specialist nurses and was characterized by the belief in the need for a hierarchy within a team and a clear leader. In contrast to this a more integrative philosophy was identified in which team members saw collaborative working and being a team player as central to cross-professional teamworking. Members understood the importance and complexity of communication and the need for effective discussion; a philosophy often held by therapy and social work professions. Lastly, the authors describe an elective working philosophy within certain professionals. This was demonstrated by professionals who prefer to work autonomously and refer to other professionals only when they perceive the need. Miller et al. (2001) used mismatches in these philosophies among members of the cross-professional team to explain team conflict and poor team outcomes.

Although philosophical differences are often mediated by the individual personality, these may also be linked to the different forms of professional socialization that occurs during training (Drinka and Clark, 2000). Certain professional groups are trained almost exclusively within a reductionist and scientific paradigm that contrasts with training of other professional groups in which a social and humanistic tradition is prevalent. In medical education, for instance, there is an emphasis on the former, a stress on the scientific basis of medicine to enhance professionalism. This could be viewed, however, as oversimplifying or narrowing the focus away from the overall picture of clients' needs. The education of nurses aims to develop a more holistic approach to patients, a less reductionist and more humanistic approach than the traditional medical model. Social workers can be perceived as at an even extreme position from medical education, where the values associated with the care of the client are at the very centre of social work practice. These very different systems may lead to the potential for poor communication. It is potentially resolved, not necessarily through a change in philosophy, but an understanding that other professionals have different perspectives of client care and that the contribution of each of these perspectives should be equally valued (Drinka and Clark, 2000).

Professional stereotyping

Another challenge to cross-professional working is the occurrence of professional stereotypes. Stereotypes are 'social categorical judgment(s) . . . of people in terms of their group memberships' (Turner, 1999: 26). It is seen as innately socially undesirable to hold stereotypes of the members of social groups other than one's own (the outgroup). However, stereotyping is a natural human process (Haslam et al., 2002) and one that may have both positive and negative outcomes. Positively, individuals may use their established stereotypes to guide their intergroup behaviours. This is a valid mechanism whereby people make sense of their interactions with other groups. They are a means to deal efficiently with an outgroup with a minimum expenditure of energy (Haslam et al., 2000; Haslam et al., 2002). In the health arena, stereotyping has been recognized as a factor that mediates group interaction. It is a means by which health and social care professionals are able, for example, to take short cuts and cope with the demands placed on them during their interactions with both the client and the employing organization (Kirkham et al., 2002). The generalized and often accurate views that the practitioner and his or her peers hold of a particular patient group may guide the professional in an appropriate manner when facing an individual from this patient group for the first time.

However, stereotypes may also generate false or negative expectations of another group's attitudes or behaviours. It is possible that these negative expectations of a group create a reality through a process of self-fulfilling prophecy (Hilton and Von Hippel, 1996). For example, prior perceptions that doctors are arrogant may taint future interactions with this group. If other health and social care professionals enter an inter-professional situation with these expectations in place, doctors may well begin to behave as expected. Alternatively, other professionals may misconstrue what otherwise would be interpreted as relatively benign behaviour. Further, if a professional group is faced with the stereotypes held of them by other groups, this may have an impact on their self-image and output. Negative perceptions of the public stereotyping of nursing, for example, has been thought to influence the development of a poor collective self-esteem, job satisfaction and performance in nursing professionals (Takase et al., 2002).

For successful teamworking, members of cross-professional teams need to develop or access the internal resources that will allow them to overcome negative stereotypes and appreciate how other disciplines understand, create and use knowledge. They need to have the flexibility to value other perspectives and embrace change and develop as a reflexive practitioner (Schön, 2004). They also need to understand each other's role and where the role of one professional begins and the other begins. These internal resources should be built during their pre-qualification training and topped up in post-qualifying career development (Carpenter, 1995a; Carpenter, 1995b; Carpenter and Hewstone, 1996; Hean et al., 2006).

Inter-professional learning

The need for training on cross-professional training has been recognized by the DoH in the UK, driven forward largely by the outcomes of the Bristol inquiry (DoH, 2001) and Laming reports (Department of Health, 2003). In the former inquiry into the deaths of children undergoing cardiac surgery at Bristol Royal Infirmary, it was recommended that health professionals (nurses, doctors and others) share education and training in order to improve their understanding and respect of each other's professional roles and responsibilities (DoH, 2001). While this inquiry did not make explicit the expected outcomes of learning together, or their conception of 'shared learning', they did identify a range of areas that were viewed as crucially important to the care of patients. These key areas included communication skills with colleagues and patients and teamworking skills (DoH, 2001).

The need to promote effective teamworking across organizations and professions through inter-professional education has been substantiated further by the findings of the inquiry into the death of Victoria Climbié (DoH, 2003). It recommended not only the establishment of a National Agency for Children & Families but that such an agency encourage institutions responsible for the training of doctors, nurses, teachers, police officers, and so on to include some form of joint training within their training programmes (Department of Health, 2003).

Both inquiries have identified the need for, and have led to the radical reform of, the education and training of a range of professionals to promote collaborative working focused on the patient or client (Humphris and Hean, 2004).

Terminology in cross-professional learning

As in cross-professional working, terminology around multi-professional or inter-professional learning must again be clarified. Students can learn about the role of other professionals in a uni-professional environment in which no contact or interaction with other student groups or professionals takes place. They may also learn multi-professionally where multi-professional education is defined as: 'Occasions when two or more professions learn side by side for whatever reason' (Freeth et al., 2002: 6).

Multi-professional learning often involves large numbers of students being taught together at the same time, in the same space and about the same topic. While there may be efficiency savings, Carpenter and Hewstone have indicated that 'simply putting students together in mixed classes . . . (may be) . . . unproductive' (Carpenter and Hewstone, 1996: 241).

On the other hand, inter-professional learning is defined as: 'Occasions when two of more professions learn with, from and about one another to improve collaboration and the quality of care (Freeth et al. 2002: 6).

Inter-professional learning necessitates that students learn 'with, from and about one another' (Freeth et al., 2002: 6) and in operational terms, this leads logically to a model of small group learning rather than large group didactic teaching. It is in this environment that students may be able to develop the internal resources they require to be good cross-professional team members.

Inter-agency working

The above discussion of a cross-professional team and its members largely takes place from a micro or even meso level of analysis. However, in a patient's care pathway, interactions between professionals often occur at a more macro level of work organization. Multiple agencies can be involved and both agency and professional boundaries negotiated.

Case study 4.1 Cross-professional working

The prevalence of mental health issues in the prison population (Joint Prison Service and National Health Service Executive, 1999; Reed, 2003; Department of Health, 2007) may partially be attributed to prisoners not being screened effectively for mental illness during earlier contact with the Criminal Justice System (CJS). For defendants to be effectively screened when passing through court, cooperation between the CJS and mental health services is required. One dimension of this is the transfer of information on the mental health of the defendant between services in the form of written reports. Reports follow the assessment of the defendant by the Mental Health Services (MHS) usually at the request of the court or other party. The report should enable the defendant to access the treatment they require and/or assist the sentencer in making an informed decision on an appropriate means of disposal. This dimension of inter-agency working has proved difficult in the past as might be expected of working between two public services so distinct in their expectations, priorities and working culture. In response to these difficulties, a partnership between the CJS and the MHS was formed in a region of the south-west of England and a pilot project was funded (South West Mental Health Assessment Pilot, 2007–2009) to implement a formal service level agreement (SLA) between the MHS and CJS to optimize the provision of reports.

In Case study 4.1 a host of agencies are involved in ensuring that defendants with mental health issues receive the support they require when passing through the court system, being diverted from the CJS if necessary. The courts and the MHS are two of these. Professionals in the courts (e.g. lawyers, judges and probation officers) work in partnership with those in the MHS (e.g. psychiatrists, community psychiatric nurses and psychologists).

Case study 4.1 also illustrates the distinction between multi- and inter-agency working. As in previous distinctions made between multi- and inter-professional working and learning, inter and multi-agency working refers to the level of integration in working across agency boundaries.

> Multi agency working implies more than one agency working with a client but not necessarily jointly. Multi agency working may be prompted by joint planning or simply be a form of replication, resulting from a lack of proper interagency co-ordination (Warmington et al., 2004: 14).

Interagency working, on the other hand, is where one or more agencies work together but where these working relationships are in a 'planned and formal way, rather than simply through informal networking' (Warmington et al., 2004: 14).

Case Study 4.1 is illustrative of how two services have moved from multi- to inter-agency working through the introduction of a SLA in which formalized relationships between agencies were established to optimize the provision of reports. Prior to the formalization of the relationship between agencies, informal networking between agencies meant court outcomes were well below optimum with delays in report provision, inappropriate report content and high, unanticipated costs being some of the poor outcomes of previous multi-agency interaction (Hean et al., 2008). The SLA between the CJS and the MHS means that formal arrangements now govern report provision and improved inter-agency working.

A framework to understand inter-agency working

Inter-agency working is complex and as such is difficult to manage and evaluate. A framework that has proved useful in making sense of this is that of the activity system (Engestrom, 2001).

The activity system as a framework is an evolution of sociocultural learning theory (Vygotsky, 1978). The basic tenet of the latter is that the meaning we make of an activity, or the learning that takes place during this activity, is a function not only of the individual's own cognition, ability or dedication. It is also mediated and influenced by factors external to the individual within the social world as well (Engestrom, 2001). Activity systems build on this individual level of analysis to take a more macro-level approach (Hean et al., 2009). Figures 4.1 and 4.2 (adapted from (Hopwood and McAlpine, 2007) illustrate two activity systems that are present in Case study 4.1. Figure 4.1 represents a single activity that takes place within the activity system – the CJS. Figure 4.2 represents a single activity that occurs within a second agency – the MHS.

In Figure 4.1, the subject is the person within an agency undertaking a particular activity. The objective is the purpose of this activity. In the court activity system, the subject is illustrated by a magistrate dealing with a defendant identified as having a potential mental health issue. In the interest of the defendant, and to inform sentencing (the object), the magistrate requests an assessment and report on the mental health of the defendant (the activity). In order to achieve this, the magistrate may complete a written assessment request or negotiate with legal advisers or liaison workers in court to make these requests. The latter are tools that mediate the activity. Surrounding this mediated activity are a range of other variables that may have influence. These include both the unwritten social norms and formal rules that govern the way in which the CJS function, for example, government-imposed targets that

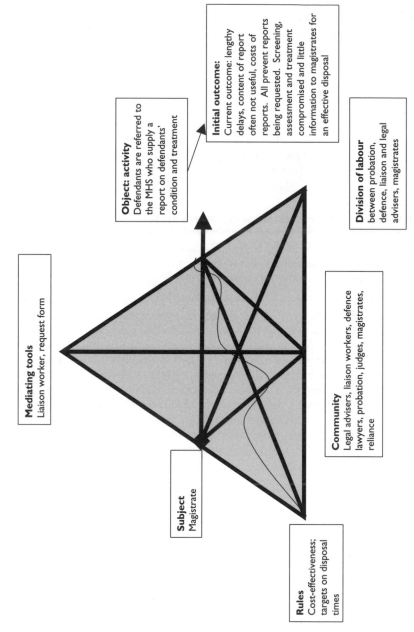

Mediating tools
Liaison worker, request form

Object: activity
Defendants are referred to the MHS who supply a report on defendants' condition and treatment

Initial outcome:
Current outcome: lengthy delays, content of report often not useful, costs of reports. All prevent reports being requested. Screening, assessment and treatment compromised and little information to magistrates for an effective disposal

Subject
Magistrate

Rules
Cost-effectiveness; targets on disposal times

Community
Legal advisers, liaison workers, defence lawyers, probation, judges, magistrates, reliance

Division of labour
between probation, defence, liaison and legal advisers, magistrates

Figure 4.1 An activity system surrounding the requests for psychiatric reports made by the CJS

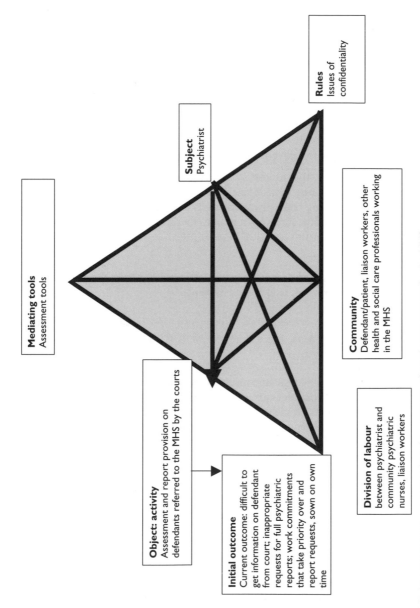

Mediating tools
Assessment tools

Subject
Psychiatrist

Rules
Issues of
confidentiality

Object: activity
Assessment and report provision on
defendants referred to the MHS by the courts

Initial outcome
Current outcome: difficult to
get information on defendant
from court; inappropriate
requests for full psychiatric
reports; work commitments
that take priority over and
report requests, sown on own
time

Community
Defendant/patient, liaison workers, other
health and social care professionals working
in the MHS

Division of labour
between psychiatrist and
community psychiatric
nurses, liaison workers

Figure 4.2 An activity system surrounding the provision of psychiatric reports by the MHS

specify the times in which court cases need to be completed. Also surrounding the activity are members of the wider CJS community who include liaison workers, defence lawyers, probation officers, court ushers, other magistrates and security personnel. Each of these members may fulfil a particular role within the CJS that will dictate how the activity under focus can be achieved (division of labour). The outcome of this activity is mediated by the complex structures that surround it. Prior to the implementation of the SLA, these outcomes were problematical caused by a range of contradictions within the activity system. For example, there is a contradiction in the activity system (Figure 4.1) between the need to request a report (object) and governing rules that stipulate that court cases need to be completed in a set time frame. As reports are often delayed, this contradiction means that magistrates were sometimes loathe to request reports as the delays the report introduces compromise the government time targets they are trying to achieve.

In Figure 4.2 the subject is a psychiatrist undertaking an assessment and making a report on a service user in contact with the CJS. The psychiatrist does this using the assessment tools available to her or him as part of their normal practice. The way in which the report is written may be underpinned by several norms and rules, for example:

- psychiatrists' view that their first responsibility is to the defendant and his or her treatment (and not punishment)
- patient confidentiality
- psychiatrists are expected to complete reports for the court on a private consultancy basis over and above their current workload.

The community that surrounds the report writing activity undertaken by the psychiatrist includes other psychiatrists, community psychiatric nurses and social workers. A clear-cut division of labour arises in report writing with psychiatrists being responsible for the full assessment and psychiatric reports required of the more seriously mentally ill or more serious offenders. Abbreviated health and social circumstance or screening reports are conducted by other health professionals. The outcomes of this activity can be challenging in that information from the courts on a patient are not easily accessible and expectations of report content and time frames are not clearly communicated (Hean et al., 2008).

In considering inter-agency working, we need to look beyond the two separate activity systems in isolation and review them in parallel, identifying how the objects of each activity are synchronous. We also need to articulate a new joint shared outcome of these two agencies working together (Figure 4.3). To optimize this joint outcome, the tensions or contradictions between the components of each system need to be identified and resolved to achieve improved joint agency outcomes (Figure 4.3). Resolutions are produced and piloted by both agencies in partnership and agencies learn together to

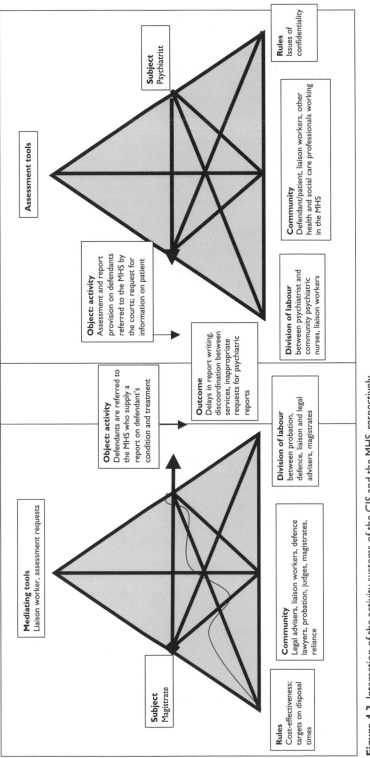

Figure 4.3 Interaction of the activity systems of the CJS and the MHS, respectively

The content within the figure:

Assessment tools

Subject Psychiatrist

Rules Issues of confidentiality

Community Defendant/patient, liaison workers, other health and social care professionals working in the MHS

Object: activity Assessment and report provision on defendants referred to the MHS by the courts; request for information on patient

Division of labour between psychiatrist and community psychiatric nurses, liaison workers

Outcome Delays in report writing, discoordination between services, inappropriate requests for psychiatric reports

Object: activity Defendants are referred to the MHS who supply a report on defendant's condition and treatment

Division of labour between probation, defence, liaison and legal advisers, magistrates

Mediating tools Liaison worker, assessment requests

Community Legal advisers, liaison workers, defence lawyers, probation, judges, magistrates, reliance

Subject Magistrate

Rules Cost-effectiveness; targets on disposal times

develop ways in which to effectively work together (Engestrom, 2001). In Case study 4.1, the mental health services and the CJS formed a working partnership to achieve just this. Representatives from each agency came together in a project steering group. The objects of each system were identified (Figures 4.1 and 4.2). Through a range of meetings between agency representatives and an evaluation of interagency challenges (Hean et al., 2008), the group identified that although they are involved in different activities, in terms of inter-agency working, they share a common overarching object – the transfer of information about a defendant with mental health issue between the two agencies. Initial joint outcomes were below optimum, the evaluation showing that there was no shared expectation of agreed timescales and that too many psychiatric reports were being requested inappropriately (Figure 4.3).

Facilitated by a project manager, contradictions within each system were identified, and a resolution put in place and tested. The jointly engineered solution was the introduction of a SLA in which the MHS are commissioned to provide 'brief screening reports' on all defendants referred to them or already known to them. These were to be done on the day or within one working day of the referral. If further information was required a health and social circumstances report or a psychiatric report would be provided to agreed timescales.

↻ Activity 4.4

Think of the service/agency in which you currently work. Use the activity system diagram to describe your service by:

- identifying a relevant subject and object
- describing the communities, rules, divisions of labour and mediating factors that surround this activity
- asking whether there are any contradictions within your system.

Now think of another service/agency with whom your service interacts. Use the activity system diagram to describe this service.

- How are your activities synchronous? Describe the joint activity you are working together to achieve.
- What are the joint outcomes of this joint activity as they now stand?
- How could these be improved?

Source: Adapted from Hopwood and McAlpine (2007)

Conclusion

This chapter has briefly introduced the concepts of multi- versus inter-professional teamworking and learning and multi- and inter-agency working.

Evidence points towards the benefits of more inter-professional working, learning and inter-agency working as key goals in practice development. However, it is clear that for a cross-professional team to work together effectively will depend on the context and objective of each individual team. We hope we have provided some insight into the issues that should be considered when thinking how to optimize the functioning of one's own cross-professional team and have provided some frameworks with which to articulate what you see in your own practice. Clarity is the first step in achieving positive action that is key to practice development.

Key points

- There are benefits to cross-professional/agency working and learning but the benefits, and ways of maximizing, vary by the purpose and context of each individual team.
- There are challenges to cross-professional/agency working including poor inter-professional stereotyping.
- It is important for practitioners to clearly articulate their practice, including that part of their practice that involves cross-professional or cross-agency working.
- The use of activity and social capital theories are tools that practitioners may find useful in this process.

Useful links

www.caipe.org.uk/
www.ihcs.bournemouth.ac.uk/etipe/who.html

References

Borrill, C., West, M., Rees, A., Dawson, J., Shapiro, D., Richards, A. et al. (2001) The Effectiveness of Health Care Teams in the National Health Service: Final Report for Department of Health. Birmingham: Aston Centre of Health Service Organisation Research (ACHSOR), University of Aston.

Borrill, C.A. and West, M. (2000) Team-working and Effectiveness in Health Care, Aston Centre of Health Service Organisation Research (ACHSOR). Birmingham: University of Aston.

Carpenter, J. (1995a) Doctors and nurses: stereotypes and stereotype change in interprofessional education, Journal of Interprofessional Care, 9(2): 151–61.

Carpenter, J. (1995b) Interprofessional education for medical and nursing students: evaluation of a programme, Medical Education, 29(4): 265–72.

Carpenter, J. and Hewstone, M. (1996) Shared learning for doctors and social workers: evaluation of a programme, British Journal of Social Work, 26(2): 239–57.

Department of Health (DoH) (2001) Learning from Bristol: The Report of the Public Inquiry into Children's Heart Surgery at the Bristol Royal Infirmary. London: Stationery Office, DoH.

Department of Health (DoH) (2003) *Victoria Climbie – Report of an Inquiry by Lord Laming*. London: Stationery Office, DoH.

Department of Health (DoH) (2007) *Improving Health, Supporting Justice*. London: DoH.

Drinka, T.J. and Clark, P. (2000) *Health Care Teamwork: Interdisciplinary Practice and Teaching*. Dover, MA: Auburn House Publishing Company.

Engestrom, Y. (2001) Expansive learning at work: toward an activity theoretical reconceptualization, *Journal of Education and Work*, 14(1): 133–56.

Eraut, M. (2003) The many meanings of theory and practice, *Learning in Health and Social Care*, 2(2): 61–5.

Freeth, D., Hammick, M., Koppel, I., Reeves, S. and Barr, H. (2002) A critical review of evaluations of interprofessional education. Working paper, Higher Education Academy, Health Sciences and Practice Network, London.

Hall, P. and Weaver, L. (2001) Interdisciplinary education and teamwork: a long and winding road, *Medical Education*, 35: 867–75.

Haslam, S.A., Powell, C. and Turner, J.C. (2000) Social identity, self-categorization, and work motivation: rethinking the contribution of the group to positive and sustainable organisational outcomes, *Applied Psychology: An International Review*, 49(3): 319.

Haslam, S.A., Turner, J.C., Oakes, P.J., Reynolds, K.J., Doosje, B. and McCarty, C. (2002) *From Personal Pictures in the Head to Collective Tools in the World: How Shared Stereotypes Allow Groups to Represent and Change Social Reality*. New York: Cambridge University Press.

Hean, S., Cowley, S., Forbes, A., Griffiths, P. and Murrells, T. (2002) *An Examination of the Potential to Identify an Instrument Reflecting Measurable Attributes of Social Capital: Final Report*. London: King's College London.

Hean, S., Craddock, D. and O'Halloran, C. (2009) Learning theories and interprofessional education: a user's guide, *Learning in Health and Social Care*, 8(4): 250–62.

Hean, S., Warr, J., Staddon, S. and Emslie, L. (2008) Challenges facing interprofessional working at the interface between the court and mental health services in the United Kingdom. Paper presented at the IAHMS Conference, Vienna, 13–17 July.

Hilton, J.L. and Von Hippel, W. (1996) Stereotypes, *Annual Review of Psychology*, 47: 237–71.

Hopwood, N. and McAlpine, L. (2007) Exploring a theoretical framework for understanding doctoral education. Paper presented at the Enhancing Higher Education, Theory and Scholarship Conference, Adelaide, Australia, 8–11 July.

Humphris, D. and Hean, S. (2004) Educating the future workforce: building the evidence about interprofessional learning, *Journal of Health Service Research Policy*, 9: 24–7.

Joint Prison Service and National Health Service Executive (1999) *The Future Organisation of Prison Health Care*. London: Department of Health (DoH).

Kirkham, M., Stapelton, H., Curtis, P. and Thomas, G. (2002) Stereotyping as a professional defence mechanism, *British Journal of Midwifery*, 10(9): 549.

Miller, C., Freeman, M. and Ross, N. (2001) *Interprofessional Practice in Health and Social Care*. London: Arnold.

Reed, J. (2003) Mental health care in prisons, *The British Journal of Psychiatry*, 182: 287–8.

Schön, D.A. (2004) *The Reflective Practitioner: How Professionals Think in Action*. New York: Basic Books.

National Health Service (NHS) Service Delivery Organization R&D (SDO) (2001) *Programme of Research on Continuity of Care*. London: NHS/SDO.

Takase, M., Kershaw, E. and Burt, L. (2002) Does public image of nurses matter? *Journal of Professional Nursing*, 18(4): 196–205.

Thylefors, I., Persson, O. and Hellstrom, D. (2005) Team types, perceived efficiency and team climate in Swedish cross-professional teamwork, *Journal of Interprofessional Care*, 19(2): 102–14.

Turner, J.C. (1999) Tome current issues in research on social identity and self categorization theories, in N. Ellemers, R. Spears and B. Doosje (eds) *Social Identity, Context, Commitment, Content*. Oxford: Blackwell Publishers, pp. 6–34.

Vygotsky, L.M. (1978) *Mind in Society*. Cambridge: Harvard University Press.

Warmington, P., Daniels, H., Edwards, A., Brown, S., Leadbetter, J., Martin, D. et al. (2004) *Interagency Collaboration: A Review of the Literature*. Bath: Learning in and for Interagency Working Project. Teaching and Learning Research Council.

5 Integrated teamworking

Kevin Stubbings, Jackie Tonkin and Rob McSherry

Introduction

Integrated teamworking is imperative in providing excellence in practice because of its associations with collaboration, partnership working, team building and dynamics, and shared working relationships to name but a few. Integrated teamworking is currently placed high on the political agenda because of media and published reports showing serious untoward incident and events when things between and across teams, disciplines, organizations and services have not worked efficiently and effectively. The importance integrated teamworking plays in supporting teams and individuals striving towards achieving excellence in practice is detailed.

The chapter highlights the drivers for integrated teamworking, defines what integrated teamworking means and involves along with highlighting the core values required by individuals and the collective team for integrated teamworking to work effectively. Examples of how integrated teamworking can be enhanced through service user and staff involvement are provided. The importance of building effective teams and teamworking is detailed along with offering a framework depicting the core factors associated with integrated teamworking. Finally, a section highlighting what it means to work in an 'integrated' way is provided.

Background

The UK health and social care systems have witnessed the introduction of a wide range and diverse set of major government policies advocating integrated teamworking. Policies include: *Care Services Improvement Partnership* (DoH 2005), *Everybody's Business* (DoH, 2006b), *National Service Framework for Mental Health* (DoH 1999), *Every Child Matters* (DoH, 2008), *Modernising Social Services Promoting Independence, Improving Protection* (DoH 1998), *Our Health our Care our Say* (DoH, 2006a) to name but a few.

The critics and cynics of health and social care policy and reform purporting integrated teamworking could argue that the government is attempting to offset the growing media reports and images highlighting spiralling costs for care, poor quality, dissatisfactions/complaints with care and treatment, system failures and blunders. The optimists and advocates of integrated teamworking may suggest that the primary aim of integrated teamworking is in enhancing the quality of care and services for all in society, offering openness, honesty and transparency around services, making professionals and workers more accountable for their practices, improving the efficiency and effectiveness of the service and improved working environments for health and social care professionals. So, in addition to policy and reform and the growing media interest in health and social care practices, what are the key drivers for integrated teamworking?

Drivers for integrated teamworking

The drivers for integrated teamworking arise from a vast and varied combination of political, professional and societal factors as outlined in Box 5.1.

Box 5.1 Drivers for integrated teamworking in health and social care

- **Nationally driven targets**: for example, dementia care strategy, end-of-life care strategy, national service frameworks
- **New ways of working**: expert patient programme, choice and patient empowerment agenda, equality and diversity agenda
- **Demography**: numbers of people requiring care exceed the numbers available to care for them (baby boom 1940–1960 and baby decline 1980)
- **Care decision tools**: for example, care pathways
- **Community verses inpatient care**: community care focus and inpatient bed reduction policies/downsizing of organizations.
- **Patient safety agenda**: learning the lessons from health and social care failings
- **Infection control agenda**: reduction of health care acquired infections.
- **Problem-focused care**: requiring a multi-agency approach; for example, falls management
- **Evidence-based/evidence-informed health and social care**: NICE guidelines
- **Terminology confusion**: confusions over existing terminology and meaning; for example, joined-up services, patient-centred care, seamlessness and partnerships. Are these something different or do they all mean the same thing?
- **New roles and new ways of working**: agenda for change, community modern matrons, physical health care practitioners, nutritional practitioners

To address and respond to the growing pressures surrounding supply and demand to innovate, change, reform or modernize health and social care as illustrated in Box 5.1, McSherry et al. (2009) suggest that it is imperative health and social care professionals understand the what, why and how integrated teamworking can support enhancing the workings of the organization. For this to occur it is essential to explore what integrated teamworking means.

What is integrated teamworking?

Activity 5.1 Reflective question

Write down what you understand by the term integrated teamworking.

Read on and compare your answers with the rest of the chapter.

The popularity of the terms 'integrated teamworking', 'integrated working' and/or 'integrated care' has as become a European and worldwide concern. This is because 'integration' or 'integrated', according Kodner and Spreeuwenberg (2002) and Grone and Garcia-Barbero (2001), is regarded as a major factor in health and social care organizations in improving performance and outcomes for individuals and teams including users of the service. Grone and Garcia-Barbero (2001) indicate that improving health and social care performance and outcomes is imperative by integrating primary, secondary and tertiary services that are often weak culminating with poor quality, inefficient and ineffective services and unnecessary inconvenience(s) to service users and carers. The World Health Organization (WHO) (1999) 'Health for All Policy Framework' identifies and acknowledges the issues surrounding integrated working by stating that 'countries should have family health physicians and nurses working at the core of this integrated primary health care service, using multi-professional teams for health, social and other sectors and involving local communities; countries should have health services that ensure individuals' participation and recognises and supports people as producers of health care'.

Given the fact that the WHO (1999) highlighted the importance of integrating services, it is not surprising that a plethora of approaches have emerged espousing to enhance integrated working of health and social care systems. Shared care, seamless care, integrated care pathways, intermediate care and continuous quality improvement are to name but a few.

Integration, as suggested by Grone and Garcia-Barbero (2001: 7), is 'the act of making a whole out of parts; the co-ordination of different activities to ensure harmonious functioning'. Integration, as highlighted in Chapter 3, is 'at the heart of whole systems approaches and, therefore, central to organizational design and performance' (Kodner and Spreeuwenberg, 2002: 2). An integrated team, according to Day (2006), is associated with inter-professional working and the way teams work: 'The greater the degree of integration, then the closer the working relationship between the different professions within the team will be' (Day, 2006: 45). What is evident from trying to define and establish what integration is and involves is the fact that the term has a wide range of meaning for different people, settings and organizations. 'This lack of conceptual clarity stands as a major barrier to promoting integrated care in both theory and practice' (Kodner and Spreeuwenberg, 2002: 1) and will ultimately influence the way services are commissioned and evaluated.

By reviewing the works of Grone and Garica-Berbero (2001), Kodner and Spreeuwenberg (2002) and Day (2006), integrated teamworking could be summarized as 'the joint working of health and social care professionals to ensure the provision of accessible, seamless services for people when required'. Furthermore, could integrated teamworking be applied to represent a team, and or service, or both? Do people actually sit together in the same office or do they attend each other's or one single multidisciplinary team? Do they use one recording system? Do they have one common point of referral or access to service? These and many more questions arise as a consequence of exploring what integrated teamworking is and involves.

A common denominator of integrated teamworking based on our experience is dependent on the application of the V framework in Table 5.1.

Table 5.1 V framework for integrated teamworking

Vision integration	Vision speaks of what integration can look like
Variation of integration	Variation speaks of a responsive robust and rigorous service design
Viability of integration	Viability asks how we keep this method alive against a constantly changing economic and political agenda

Table 5.1 highlights how and why integrated teamworking is dependent on vision, variation and viability. The V framework recognizes that the vision will be influenced by the location and has seen the variation that is needed to sustain a viable service. For example, developing integrated teamworking in a large rural area will not be the same as a large urban conurbation would require. By acknowledging these differences and challenges, the obstacles to integrated teamworking can be overcome. Although throughout the integration process evaluation of the effectiveness of the various stages in promoting the core values of integrated teamworking is crucial. So what are the core values associated with integrated teamworking?

The core values of integrated teamworking

High-quality health and social care depends on health, social and primary care professionals working and communicating effectively together; it is no more complex than that nor should it be. However, there are some core values that promote effective integrated teamworking and communication. Working within and with teams using a practice development framework (PDF) like those highlighted by Manley et al. (2008) and McSherry and Warr (2008, 2006) recognizes that successful integrated teams have a core element for success.

The perfect combination and harmony of simple elements are as follows:

Having a vision: are all members of the team aware of the vision and what you are trying to achieve?

Sharing the vision: has the opportunity to share the vision among all the team members and stakeholders occurred in order to encourage signing up and engagement?

Encouraging involvement: what strategies have been developed and deployed to encourage participation within the team and in seeking to work together?

Supporting innovation and change: is the team supported by leaders and managers, as highlighted in Chapter 2, to work together?

Enthusiasm: does the team have sufficient members who are eager to pursue the team's vision through the challenges associated with working between and across teams?

Communication: has a communication strategy been developed to support the team's sharing of the vision and progression internally and externally to the team?

Collaboration: as part of the team's strategy, has any consultation been planned to establish key stakeholders' views and opinions and how they may become integral to the team?

Celebration: what systems and processes have been developed to celebrate when things go well or indeed to learn from when things do not go as planned?

Adopting a PDF is ideal in fostering integrated working because it:

> draws on many different and diverse disciplines, which in turn enables all professional functions to be integrated for the benefit of patients. It is a prerequisite to clinical effectiveness, continuous quality improvement, and the development of a culture that facilitates the responsive and pro-active action necessary for effective healthcare (McCormack and Manley, 2003: 23).

The success to integrated teamworking is the establishment of a systematic robust framework for your team and/or organization to utilize so that it can be replicated and repeated by anyone with a degree of capability, but which will guarantee a quality product each time. Eventually, experience (both positive and negative) will inform you to adapt or refine the framework to make it unique to your requirements but you will always need the core elements, as highlighted above. Howarth et al. (2006) recognize that health and social care professionals need to develop skills in practice development if they are to effectively support integrated working and to achieve this requires organizations to allow staff to be creative, intuitive, empowered and be supported to take positive risks.

Similarly to Howarth et al. (2006), works by Hudson (2006a) and Coxon (2005) highlight the significance of health and social care professionals having sound awareness of how as part of their role and responsibility they can enable or hinder practice innovation and enhancements. The works by Hudson (2006a) and Coxon (2005) focus on the experiences of professional health care workers and factors that either support or restrain good integrated working. A limitation of Coxon's (2005) work over Hudson (2006a) is the lack of focus on the experience of the service user/carer or by offering an evaluation of effective practice from a range of perspectives; a concern echoed by Kodner and Spreeuwenberg (2002: 3):

> professionals seldom look at the world of health care through the patient lens. This is not surprising. Traditionally, caregivers demand that their patient be compliant, therefore, usually do not expect that their concerns will come first, or even be seriously addressed. This attitude, though challenging, has permeated health care until now.

Whichever term we use to reflect integrated teamworking and practice development, the perspective should prioritize that of the service user/carer and the focus should be on providing evidence of quality patient-related outcomes through integrated teamworking. A method for developing and evaluating service user and carer outcomes is through service user and carer storytelling (Box 5.2).

Box 5.2 Service user and carer storytelling

Storytelling 'has long been appreciated as an art form and as a way for a culture to convey and recreate learning from generation to generation' (Restrepo and Davis, 2003: 43). The premise behind storytelling, according to Hill Bailey and Tilley (2002: 575), is the 'belief that individuals make sense of their world most effectively by telling stories' that offer an ideal medium for the sharing and learning through and from experiences.

Service user and carer storytelling involves an informal interview process using a semi-structured questionnaire. Service users and carers are encouraged to share their journey or experience from whichever point they choose. The facilitator has a key role in being able to actively listen and reflect the key messages, emotions, values and beliefs and learning from the story.

Storytelling is a very powerful testimony of the care journey offering valuable insight into individual experiences and the effects that services, working styles and individual capability can have on providing a person-centred care. Ultimately, storytelling provides 'access to subjective reality, that is *their truth*, and the meanings of their experiences, which are vitally important for understanding of and for providing appropriate care' (Hill Bailey and Tilley (2002: 581, authors' emphasis).

Storytelling

Offering quality patient-related outcomes associated with integrating teamworking are dependent on awareness raising, sharing, implementation and evaluation of core values. The core values associated with integrated teamworking are a combination and harmonization of having a vision, sharing the vision, encouraging involvement, supporting innovation and change, enthusiasm, communication, collaboration and celebration. It is also important to look not just at integrated team or service distinctions but also at the distinctions made between multi-professional and integrated working. Masterson (2002) argues that multi-professional work is seen as a cooperative enterprise in which traditional forms and divisions of professional knowledge and authority are retained. Inter-professional work is having a willingness to share and give up exclusive claims to specialized knowledge and authority if other professional groups can meet patient/client needs more efficiently and appropriately. So what are the core factors associated with integrated teamworking?

Core factors of integrated teamworking: a framework for excellence in practice

> ↻ **Activity 5.2 Integrated teamworking in action**
>
> • Considering your own organization, who do you see as the people who work within an integrated team?
> • Reflect on what skills you feel these people use that promote effective integrated team working.
>
> Read on and compare your answers with the rest of the chapter.

Integrated teamworking or integrated care, as suggested by Grone and Garcia-Barbero (2001), is challenging because of the difficulty in uniting the various parts that constitutes the 'health [social care] system – functions, institutions, and professions in order to improve the performance of the health [social care] system' (Grone and Garcia-Barbero 2001: 1). For integrated teamworking to occur effectively McCallin (2001), Kodner and Spreeuwenberg (2002), Webster (2002), Brown et al. (2003) and Cashman et al. (2004) highlight that building effective teams and teamworking is imperative.

Building effective teams and teamworking

The terms 'teams' and 'teamwork[ing],' as argued McCallin (2001), are often used interchangeably, which renders them vague. Teams, as suggested by Manion et al. 2001: 422 are:

> a small number of consistent people committed to a relevant shared purpose, with common performance goals, complementary and over lapping skills, and a common approach to work. Team members hold themselves mutually accountable for the team's results and outcomes.

Team*working* however is associated with how the team works collectively, cooperatively, consistently and effectively in communicating, assimilating and evaluating performance in achieving the shared purpose, goals and common approach to service delivery. Adopting an effective team and teamworking approach is imperative for integrated teamworking to occur.

Optimism and pessimism

Hudson (2006a, 2006b) developed two models, which he termed 'optimistic' and 'pessimistic', for understanding the factors that may underpin the different rates of inter-professional achievement. Historically, professionals tend to focus on the factors that divide them, or make them unique as a profession. While these factors are important, more so, professionals are recognizing the factors they have in common, and more often these outweigh the factors of uniqueness.

Being the pessimist only enables us to focus on the barriers to integration where what is required is for us to be optimistic and seek out the things we have in common and to cease the opportunities for attuning to service user and carer values.

In the spirit of fostering an integrated approach to organizational working, we approach highlighting our experiences in an integrated way. Coming from senior nursing and social work backgrounds, we are now working in partnership within a large National Health Service (NHS) Foundation Trust specializing in mental health services (MHS). We have seen integration begin, blossom, boom and then be pruned, and re-emerge in another form, so know the highs, lows and pitfalls of the process. For integrated teamworking to occur from our experiences, we have identified eight core factors to effective integrated teamworking: creative leadership, team comfort and compassion, team climate, team caring, team common language, team combustion, team champagne and cork and team common sense.

Figure 5.1 offers a framework for integrated working in health and social care by focusing attention on practice development 'centred on promoting patient-centeredness through the utilisation of a facilitative approach to team working, collaboration and partnership building' (McSherry and Warr, 2008: 3). Furthermore, Manley et al. (2008: 9) suggest that the 'learning that occurs brings about transformations of individual and team practices. This is sustained by embedding both processes and outcomes in corporate strategy', thus highlighting the importance of personal and professional development within the organization along with paying attention to personal values, attitude and beliefs of those working in the team. The factors supporting or restraining integrated teamworking are derived from what professionals have described as a common language towards achieving integrated teamworking and are detailed below. Finally, the ultimate goal of integrated teamworking is the provision of quality patient-related outcomes for users

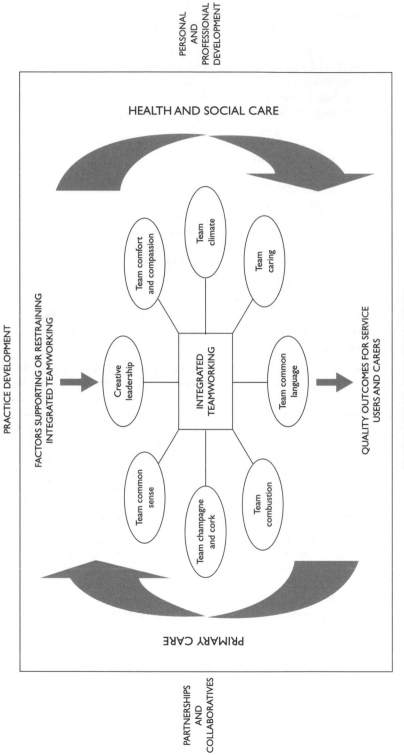

Figure 5.1 A framework for integrated working in health and social care

and carers along with enhanced communication, shared working, an understanding of complementary points of view, supportive working environment and enhanced productivity and outcomes for the team.

Creative leadership

As already highlighted in Chapter 2, leadership is fundamental to ensuring quality along with integrated teamworking. Effective creative leadership is central to the success of any integrated team; this is a key gatekeeping role that requires the individual to demonstrate capability whatever the professional background. Covey (1992) relates to the leader knowing themselves before embarking on knowing others. Therefore, the person designated leader of the team has to be self-aware and be attuned to their own leadership capability and to able to transfer these skills into practice; alongside self-awareness the leader needs to understand what their core value and belief system is and, how this can influence and alienate others. Leadership style needs to reflect a balance of transformational and transactional traits and the leader needs to be comfortable with empowering others and to nurture the creativity within the team. The ability for the leader to set clear goals and to give positive feedback is a critical success factor. Bandura and Cervone (1986) suggest control is exercised through the team's respect of the leader's quality and style, combined with a robust knowledge base and the ability to create, develop and share a clear vision for the team and align them to it. Teams that are purely managed and not led will never work effectively in an integrated way.

Team comfort and compassion

Team comfort and compassion is borne out of mutual respect and understanding for each other's personal, social and professional background (training and education, etc.) roles and responsibilities within the team, cultural background and how this conflicts or is enhanced by the organizational culture. Team comfort and compassion reflects the core values of reciprocity, open mindedness, fairness, flexibility, attentive listening and shared governance. Team comfort and compassion is essential in that teams have a healthy working organizational environment in which to disagree, debate and agree common solutions that require consistency of approach. Ethical approaches tend to move from traditional deontological or teleological approaches to reflect more value and belief-driven ethics, person centeredness, equality and diversity. The team needs to be tolerant and forgiving in nature that relies heavily on the operational policies underpinning the team and service structure, the team work ethic and vision.

Team climate

Team climate reflects the changing working environment and organization we live and work within; for example, the changing demographics of client groups, changing pressures in society impacting on health and well-being, changing developments with the health and social care field, changing attitudes and expectations of professionals and service users and carer's expectation. Team climate recognizes the above challenges of integrated teamworking and how through adopting the approach it is trying to avoid being a service which is all things to all men/women. Team climate tends to accommodate the fluctuation between periods of relative stability then rapid change offering solutions by attempting to have a joined service and joined-up thinking between the professionals for the common vision, goals, and objectives for the team.

Team caring

Caring involves getting the essentials right and involves the core values of genuineness, empathy and validation (not necessarily agreeing but acknowledgement of someone's feelings and how those emotions affect that person). Team caring relates to the conscious self; for example, not expecting others to do things for you but to pull equal weight within the team not just in workload but in generating ideas and creativity. The outcomes for users, carers and staff matter. Team caring is not just a case of feeding the corporate beast for volume, figures, targets and league tables but requires team members to have a core range of personal and interpersonal skills that both compliment and are an asset to the team. Put the wrong ingredient in the cake and chaos ensues. The core qualities akin to team caring relate to interpersonal skills, verbal and non-verbal skills, negotiation and problem-solving skills, reflective practitioner and self-awareness. Team caring also relates to staff commitment to the concept of integrated teamworking.

Team common language

Team common language is associated with the use of terminology and phraseology within the team to reflect all disciplines and the prevention of isolation of one or more groups. Team common language relies on terms that do not isolate one professional group and avoids misinterpretation or double meaning. Team common language relates to the wider concepts of having co-proximity and location, information technology links and access, particularly if staff are operating between several electronic systems that do not talk to each other. Team common language links to the joint management and pooling of budgets and resources, shared governance arrangements, conflict resolution, inter-professional learning and practice/education and open sharing of knowledge and skills.

Team combustion

Team combustion reflects the notion that integrated teams are usually relatively small teams therefore there is often an expectation that they will absorb everything that is thrown at them. But to prevent this dilution and potential in effectiveness, the team needs to consider a whole systems approach that involves quality:

- clinical supervision
- team/performance supervision (you could introduce the concept of team appraisal here over individual appraisal)
- caseload management systems and supervision
- referral processes
- work allocation systems
- not replacing like for like – new ways of working agenda, what does the team really need to make it more effective?
- informal supervision systems and recognizing the value of these

Team champagne and cork

Team champagne and cork relates to harnessing the creativity within the team through a PDF. The process of assessment and benchmarking of the team against a range of standards to allow them to focus on action planning (relates to the Tiger Woods analogy; i.e., the pursuit at being the best at what you do and what it takes to get there, constantly reshaping and improving to set the benchmark for others to follow) where successful teams do not fear this process, they embrace it. Team champagne and cork relates to how teams celebrate their success (or not as is often the case) and recognizes the skills and development/support needed for the team to move on to the next level. To achieve team champagne and cork requires strong organizational and managerial/leader commitment; hence, once the cork is pulled and the champagne starts to flow, you would not be the one trying to stem it and put the cork back in, it is counterproductive and a quality product is wasted. 'Once people get a taste for champagne there is hopefully no going back to cheap wine!'

Team common sense

Team common sense relates to equity in terms and conditions, opportunities for development, leading change and evaluating service improvement, mutual respect and appreciation, compromise and taking risks and not being afraid to fail. The difference is that good teams know why they failed before they move on to the next solution. Being realistic in what teams and individuals are capable of achieving and recognizing stress factors and disharmony within teams are all imperative to having sound team common sense. Team common sense should be viewed as part of any model/framework of continuous quality improvement and pursuit of excellence in practice.

Having offered a case study illustrating a possible framework for promoting integrated teamworking, it is important to highlight what it means to work in an integrated way.

What does it mean to work in an 'integrated' way?

To be part of a team that works in a truly integrated manner can mean many things. Perhaps the best measure is that such a team cannot easily be identified! The reason for this is the collaborative working should be seamless and the individual receiving services should find the experience so inclusive that they do not actually know that both health and social resources are being made available to them. This may sound idealistic but it can and does happen. An assessment can be made by a member of an integrated service and from that assessment both further health-based services can be activated, and any social care needs set up. For example, community-based home care services provided by the local authority can be requested and the social care provider will accept the care plan from whichever professional regardless of their 'employer'. Rather than undertaking a reassessment the integrated team will be aware of these requirements and have protocols in place to meet the local authority rules and charging policies.

In order for service users to move through the service feeling understood, it is the number of times the same information is requested that can often indicate the true level of collaborative working! It is a source of frustration to all of us to be asked over and over again for the same details. While the need to double-check to ensure the correct identity of an individual is best practice in many situations, we need to ensure that other best practice standards are not lost because this element is allowed to dominate. Often we find that having established a person's identity, practitioners go on to ask routine questions almost by rote! Please do not misunderstand us around this point. Establishing this type of information is crucial. However, it forms only part of an assessment and communicating with people in a way that reflects a shared awareness and by avoiding duplication of effort will often build that person's confidence that the team understands their situation.

Team confidence

For a team to work efficiently and effectively in an integrated way requires total confidence in each other to deliver the best result; therefore, focusing on ensuring team confidence is essential. The best results depend on having a clear goal where more than one team member is usually required to achieve it where all share in the result whether this is good or not so good!

Collaboration between members of a multidisciplinary team can mean that initial assessments are undertaken often by two team members from any discipline and the outcomes shared with other members of the team if services are identified. This saves time and leads to a confidence among the team that each profession is valued and none is dominant.

Team capability

For your team to be capable of working and responding in an integrated way requires individuals to have a combination of personal and professional qualities as highlighted in Box 5.3.

Box 5.3 Qualities akin to integrated teamworking

Personal	Professional
• Open	• Competent
• Genuine	• Capable
• Empathic	• Motivated
• Trustworthy	• Respected
• Self-aware	• Empowering
• Confident	• Enabling
• Motivated	• Pro-transformation

Box 5.3 highlights the important fact that capacity within the team is dependent on the team members having a combination of the various qualities to work efficiently and effectively together. For example, designated crisis response workers are virtually unknown within older people services although older people do have crises; these are usually addressed within the community mental health team and can affect capacity to take on new referrals. Truly integrated teams often find it easier to react to these situations as there is a flexibility around allocation of assessments, it is not always essential for the community psychiatric nurse to undertake the initial visit, that can be done by the social worker and occupational therapist. Within an integrated team, it is about ensuring the best person responds to a particular crisis or situation in maximizing the resources.

Conclusion

A plethora of terms around this subject can be found but do they all mean the same thing? For teams to work in a truly integrated way value needs to be added to the process. Truly integrated teams demonstrate this value along with the vision for the service user/person/patient to experience a pathway that reflects the interventions required without needing a multitude of 'services' being identified. Integrated teams welcome scrutiny and embrace the concept of practice development in the pursuit of excellence. To sum it all up, the heart of an integrated team is the person-centred focus and the flexibility that this truly requires. Integrated teamworking is imperative if excellence in practice is to become a reality rather than a myth. It would be fantastic in the future if integrated teamworking and service provision became the norm and not the desirable as is often the case within health and social care organizations. For excellence in practice to occur, it is important to direct attention on teamworking, team dynamics and roles and responsibilities within and between the team members of the collective service(s). For effective integrated teamworking to occur, both integrated services and teams should not become complacent and/or take this for granted but seek to work in an even more 'integrated' fashion with other stakeholders and partners in the future.

Key points

- The UK health and social care systems have witnessed the introduction of a wide range and diverse set of major government policies advocating integrated teamworking.
- The drivers for integrated teamworking arise from a vast and varied combination of political, professional and societal factors.
- It is imperative that health and social care professionals understand the what, why and how integrated teamworking can support enhancing the workings of the organization.
- The popularity of the terms 'integrated teamworking', 'integrated working' and/or 'integrated care' has become a European and worldwide concern.
- Integrated teamworking could be summarized as 'the joint working of health and social care professionals to ensure the provision of accessible, seamless services for people when required'.
- High-quality health and social care depends on health, social and primary care professionals working and communicating effectively together; it is no more complex than that nor should it be.
- The success of integrated teamworking is the establishment of a recipe for your team and/or organization so that it can be replicated and repeated by anyone with a degree of capability; an approach that will hopefully guarantee a quality experience and outcome each time.
- Offering quality patient-related outcomes associated with integrated teamworking are dependent on awareness raising, sharing, implementation and evaluation of core values. The core values associated with integrated teamworking are a combination and harmonization of having a vision, sharing the vision, encouraging involvement, supporting innovation and change, enthusiasm, communication, collaboration and celebration.

- The ultimate goal of integrated teamworking is the provision of quality patient-related outcomes for users and carers along with enhanced communication, shared working, an understanding of complementary points of view, supportive working environment and enhanced productivity and outcomes for the team.
- To be part of a team that works in a truly integrated manner can mean many things. Perhaps the best measure is that such a team cannot easily be identified!

Useful links

International Journal of Integrated Care. Available online at www.ijic.org/index.html (accessed November 2009).

References

Bandura, A. and Cervone, D. (1986) Differential engagement of self-reactive influences in cognitive motivation, *Organizational Behavior and Human Decision Processes*, 38: 92–113.

Brown, L., Tucker, C. and Domokos, T. (2003) Evaluating the impact of integrated health and social care teams on older people living in the community, *Health and Social Care in the Community*, 11(2): 85–94.

Cashman, B.S., Reidy, P., Cody, K. and Lemay, C.A. (2004) Developing and measuring progress toward collaborative, integrated, interdisciplinary health care teams, *Journal of Interprofessional Care*, 18(2): 183–96.

Covey, S. (1992) *The 7 Habits of Highly Effective People.* London: Simon & Schuster UK Ltd.

Coxon, K. (2005) Common experiences of staff working in integrated health and social care organisations: a European perspective, *Journal of Integrated Care*, 13(2): 13–21.

Day, J. (2006) Interprofessional working, in L. Wigens (ed.) *Expanding Nursing and Health Care Practice Series.* Cheltenham: Nelson Thornes.

Department of Health (DoH) (1998) *Modernising Social Services Promoting Independence, Improving Protection.* London: HMSO.

Department of Health (1999) *National Service Framework for Mental Health.* London: HMSO.

Department of Health (2005) Care *Services Improvement Partnership.* London: HMSO.

Department of Health (2006a) *Our Health our Care our Say.* London: HMSO.

Department of Health (2006b) *Everybody's Business.* London: HMSO.

Department of Health (2008) *Every Child Matters.* London: HMSO.

Grone, O. and Garcia-Barbero, M. (2001) Integrated care: a position paper of the WHO European office for integrated health care services, *International Journal of Integrated Care*, 1(1): 1–10.

Hill Bailey, P. and Tilley, S. (2002) Storytelling and the interpretation of meaning in qualitative research, *Journal of Advanced Nursing*, 38(6): 574–83.

Howarth, M., Holland, K., Maria, J. and Grant, J.M. (2006) Integrative literature review and meta-analysis education needs for integrated care: a literature review, *Journal of Advanced Nursing*, 56(2): 144–56.

Hudson, B. (2006a) Integrated team working: you can get it if you really want it: part I, *Journal of Integrated Care*, 1(14): 13–21.

Hudson, B. (2006b) Integrated team working: part II: making the inter-agency connections, *Journal of Integrated Care*, 2(14): 26–36.

Kodner, L.D. and Spreeuwenberg, C. (2002) Integrated care: meaning, logic, applications, and implications – a discussion paper, *International Journal of Integrated Care*, 2(14): 1–6.

McCallin, A. (2001) Interdisciplinary practice – a matter of teamwork: an integrated literature review, in J. Manion, W. Lorimer and W.J. Leander, (eds) *Team-based Health Care Organisations: Blueprint for Success*. Aspen, CO: Gaithersburg.

Manion, J., Lorimer, W. and Leander, W.J. (1996) *Team-based Health care Organizations. Blueprint for Success*. Aspen, M.D.

Manley, K., McCormack, B. and Wilson, V. (2008) *International Practice Development in Nursing and Healthcare*. Oxford: Blackwell Publishing.

Masterton, A. (2002) Cross-boundary working: a macro-political analysis of the impact on professional roles, *Journal of Clinical Nursing*, 11(3): 331–9.

McCallin, A. (2001) Interdisciplinary practice: a matter of teamwork: an integrated literature review, *Journal of Clinical Nursing*, 10: 419–28.

McCormack, B. and Manley, K. (2003) Practice development: purpose, methodology, facilitation and evaluation, *Nursing in Critical Care*, 8(1): 22–9.

McSherry, R., Scott, K. and Farlow, S. (2009) Practice development, in F. Timmins, and C. McCabe (eds) *Day Surgery Contemporary Approaches to Nursing Care*. Chichester: Wiley-Blackwell.

McSherry, R. and Warr, J. (2008) *An Introduction to Excellence in Practice Development in Health and Social Care*. Maidenhead: Open University Press.

McSherry, R. and Warr, J. (2006) Practice development: confirming the existence of a knowledge and evidence base, *Practice Development in Health Care*, 5(2): 55–79.

Restrepo, E. and Davis, L. (2003) Storytelling: both art and therapeutic practice, *International Journal of Human Caring*, 7(1): 43–8.

Webster, J. (2002) Teamwork: understanding multi-professional working, *Nursing Older People*, 14(3): 14–19.

World Health Organization (WHO) (1999) *Health 21: The Health for All Policy Framework for the WHO European Region*. (European Health for All Series No. 6). Copenhagen: WHO.

6 | Factors influencing collaborative working

Rob McSherry

Introduction

This chapter briefly outlines the enabling and inhibiting factors influencing collaborative working within health and social care at an individual, team and organizational level in the quest for excellence in practice. It outlines what the key enablers and inhibitors are and how they may be challenged, overcome and resolved in the pursuit for excellence in practice. This is achieved by exploring the enablers and inhibitors to collaborative working associated with culture, management, leadership, communication, education and training, knowledge, support and resources.

Background

Collaborative working according to Chesterman (2001: 778) is not a new concept: 'human beings first started collaborating in search for food. We have had several millennia to work out how to do it. So in one sense it is somewhat strange that in the twenty-first century we find that "partnerships are good in theory but incredibly difficult in practice" '.

Collaborative working as suggested by the National Health Service (NHS) Institute for Innovation and Improvement (2009: 1) is about 'being committed to working and engaging constructively with internal and external stakeholders'. It is important because collaboration:

> is critical in delivering measurable and radical health [and social care] improvements in a complex and changing health and social care environment. Effective partnership promotes the sharing of information and appropriate prioritisation of limited resources. It also supports 'joined up' provision of integrated care (NHS Institute for Innovation and Improvement (2009: 1).

Collaboration is defined by Collins (1987: 170) as 'to work together; in some literary, artistic, or scientific undertaking; to cooperate with an enemy invader' rendering the term according to Callagan (2006: 389) almost difficult to define and apply to the health and social care context. However, further exploration of Collins' (1987) definition of collaboration offers some useful insights associated with enablers and inhibitors to excellence in practice.

First, excellence in practice warrants effective integrated teamworking through building genuine working relationships and partnerships within and between team members and teams, communication and the sharing of information.

Second, excellence in practice is founded on fostering a creative innovative culture and working environment that embraces the challenge associated with change where communications and artistic creativity and/or science are maximized.

Third, resolving conflicts of interest, between professional groups and disciplines through building bridges, between individuals, teams, organizations and between and within teams and professional disciplines is imperative. The fostering of shared working relationships and responsibilities where dominant groups or an individual are excluding innovation and change through encouraging participation is essential.

Fourth, the notion of challenging and developing a commitment to innovate through avoiding the imposing of views that have a tendency to oppress and stifle participation is a key ingredient to effective collaborative working.

Finally, for some health and social care organizations, teams and professionals, the issues affecting collaborative working are not directly associated with what collaborative working is or involves, but in resolving the inhibitors, obstacles or barriers associated with the demands on busy individuals and teams working within and between the various ward, units, departments and/or centres associated with fostering collaborative working.

The enabling and inhibiting influencing collaborative working

The general definition for the term/phrase 'inhibit' or 'inhibitor' is 'to hold back or keep from some action' (Collins 1987: 442). Enable or enabler is 'to make able; provide with means, opportunity, power, to do something' (Collins 1987: 284).

Activity 6.1   Establishing the enablers and inhibitors to collaborative working

Write down what you think are the potential enablers and inhibitors to collaborative working in your area of practice.

Read on and compare your answers with the rest of the chapter.

Collins' (1987) definition of enablers and inhibitors offers a useful insight into understanding the challenges associated with fostering, implementing and evaluating the relative merits and demerits of collaborative working within health and social care.

First, 'to hold back' is highly significant to collaborative working. Holding back or withholding something may create an obstruction to the sharing of information, creating a vision, communicating team objectives, encouraging and engaging the team with the innovation and change factors that are highly important to fostering a culture and working environment founded on collaborative working. An inhibitor to collaborative working could therefore be regarded as an obstruction related to anything that affects the quality of the vast array of systems and processes akin to an individual and or team structure(s); for example, an obstruction in the channels of communication and information-giving between health and social care professionals and patients/users about preoperative risks and benefits associated with a certain procedure; or the failure to document an incident in the patient's health or social care records after a fall, where the patient/family complain about the incident asking for a full explanation several weeks after the event and no one can remember the event.

Second, 'keep from some action' is again highly important to nurturing collaborative working suggesting the need for dividing or keeping something apart for a specific purpose, whether this be for an intentional and/or unintentional reason. For example, a team member avoids attending a mutidisciplinary team meeting because of personal conflicts with other team members and non-disclosure of key information to team members or patients/carers through ineffective communication or inadequate interpersonal skills.

Enabling as suggested by Collins (1987) is a major contributing factor associated with effective collaborative working. Collaborative working is about freeing up individuals, teams and organizations, resources or availability of time so that active and not passive participation in advancing and evaluating practice is afforded to all. Enabling collaborative working is dependent on providing individuals with the means to get involved, the opportunity to participate and the power to feel included not excluded or marginalized as a team player. Enabling plays a major role in facilitating excellence in practice because 'the delivery of improved health [and social care] is increasingly dependent on the ability of diverse professions, organisations and departments to work together across conceptual and organisational boundaries' (McMurray 2006: 238). Enabling collaborative and partnership working is ultimately at the core of excellence in practice.

It is evident from Collins' (1987) definition that inhibitors can be positive and/or negative, intentional or unintentional in nature, which has immense importance when exploring the issues associated with collaborative working in health and social care. For example, collaborative working could be viewed positively at organizational level because it provides a means of improving quality by developing integrated teams, crossing professional boundaries through team building and effective teamworking and by developing associated systems and processes, but for an individual in daily practice it is viewed negatively because it is just another buzzword without relevance to their daily practices. To avoid and resolve the potential inhibitors associated with fostering a culture and working environment through collaborative working, it is important that during the implementation process individuals, the team and organization collectively sign up and embrace this approach to working with enthusiasm rather than scepticism. Collaborative working can really only be satisfactorily implemented on the basis of a welcomed initiative with the potential for developing real improvements in quality of patient care rather than a political imposition (Edwards and Packham, 1999). Collaboration and teamwork according to Hunter (1996) and Williams (2002) cited in McMurray (2006: 238) 'have become watchwords for the organisation of care. They are the preferred organisational solution to meta-issues and policy messes beyond the scope of any one agency or group'. Meta-issues in the context of collaborative working could be associated with establishing integrated teamworking that may be promoted or hampered by a combination of individual and organizational factors, which can be multiple, complex and diverse in nature.

For some health and social care organizations, teams and individual's collaborative working or partnership working is not the perceived norm. Collaborative working could be viewed as yet another buzzword, fad or preferred way of working imposed by government in response to the poor media view of the health and social care because of the high profile cases that have highlighted inadequate standards and practices associated with joint working, integrated teamworking or collaborative working. Cases like those in Box 6.1:

Box 6.1 Media health and social care cases highlighting the importance of collaborative working

Baby P

The recent Baby P case highlighted major inadequacies in the way health and social care agencies and organizations were addressing child protection policies and procedures.

Victoria Climbie

The Victoria Climbie case in 2002 highlighted major concerns associated with multi-agency working between and across health and social care professional boundaries (McSherry and Warr 2008).

Mid Staffordshire NHS Foundation Trust

The Healthcare Commission highlighted serious failings with the standards of patient care and dangerously low staffing levels and serious issues relating to how staff concerns were listened and responded to.

Harold Shipman

Following the Shipman Enquiry in 2001, a General Practitioner was convicted of the murder of 15 patients as a result of morphine poisoning (Ramsey, 2001).

Alitt Enquiry

The Alitt Enquiry where a qualified enrolled nurse working in a paediatric unit was convicted of murdering four children and injuring nine others (MacDonald, 1996).

The cases highlighted in Box 6.1 have significantly affected the public's confidence in the quality of care offered by health and social care, a confidence that requires rebuilding. Put bluntly, collaborative working offers a framework that is designed to help doctors, nurses, therapists, care workers, care managers, indeed all health and social care staff, to improve organizational, team and individual standards and quality of care. To achieve some of the many potential benefits of collaborative working through integrating teams (Box 6.2) requires a shift in attitudes and culture to a proactive and active rather than a reactive and passive one.

Box 6.2 Potential benefits of collaborative working through integrating teams

- Establishing a clear vision and goals
- Having a shared vision
- Reducing clinical risks
- Promoting continuous quality improvement
- Providing the best practices based on the best evidence
- Delivery of a multidisciplinary service by professionals who have the correct knowledge, skills and competence
- Lifelong learning

McMurray (2006: 239) indicates that we need to develop a mutual reciprocity (reciprocity referring to reciprocal relationships; mutual exchange; Collins, 1987: 704) of sharing between and within teams, groups and professional disciplines. This is because a 'reciprocity bolstered by the sharing of clients, skills and responsibilities provides an unquestionable logic to the development of collaborative working across health and social care' (Collins, 1987: 704). The continued occurrence of cases highlighted in Box 6.1 illustrating that the promise of collaborative working through integrated care is still to materialize. The 'challenge then is to understand why the great divide between health and social care persists, and ascertain whether, and by what means, the forces acting in opposition to reciprocity based partnerships might be resisted' (McMurray, 2006: 239).

The development of an effective organizational culture and working environment centres on a philosophy of shared working relationships and partnerships, learning and celebrating from things that go well and not so well. As suggested by Davies et al. (2000), it is about learning from the past to inform the future habits and develop some new habits. The perceived inhibiting factors associated with collaborative working are vast but not insurmountable, as outlined in Box 6.3.

Box 6.3 Perceived inhibiting factors associated with collaborative working

- lack of understanding
- fear
- no clear vision
- it's nothing new
- it's a passing fad
- lack of time
- lack of resources
- lack of support
- inadequate information/no information
- poor leadership
- ineffective communication.

Note: This not an exhaustive list of the potential or perceived inhibitors to collaborative working.

Box 6.3 shows that the perceived inhibiting factors surrounding collaborative working originate from a combination of either or both internal and external sources that can affect the organization, teams and individual's ability to pursue reciprocity, as illustrated in Table 6.1.

The internal and external factors affecting collaborative working relating to the organization or individual, as shown in Table 6.1, can be themed into several key areas as outlined in Figure 6.1 and discussed here.

Culture

What do we mean by culture? Culture is defined as 'the skills and arts, etc. of a given people in a given period; civilisation . . . improvements of the mind, manners, etc. development by special training or care' (Collins, 1987: 214). During the late 1990s and early 2000s the word culture has become more prominent within health and social care, perhaps as a result of the many failures of health and social care systems, processes and the high-profile professional misconduct cases, as previously mentioned. A common theme that has emerged following the inquiries outlined in Box 6.1 investigations/

Table 6.1 Internal and external factors influencing collaborative working

	Internal	External
Individual	• Knowledge • Understanding • Confidence • Ownership • Fear • Resistance to change • Communication • Information	• Support • Resources • Time • Communication • Information
Organizational	• Culture • Leadership • Ownership • Management • Communication • Information	• Political • Demand • Performance • Expectations • Resourcing

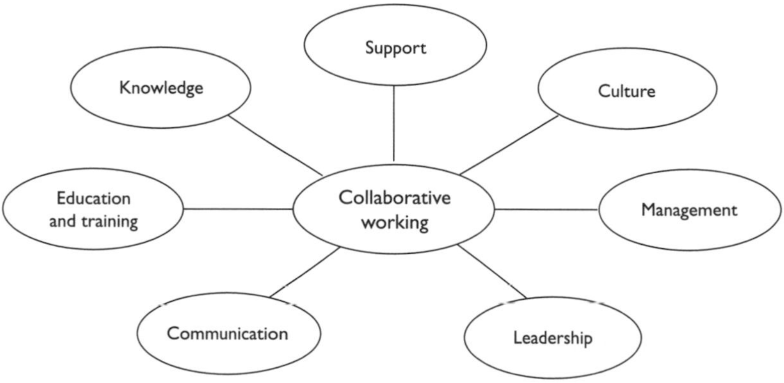

Figure 6.1 Key themes linked to fostering collaborative working

reviews is the use of the word 'culture' or phrases like 'open or closed culture'. The questions posed by some health and social care professionals are:

- Why is creating the right culture important to health and social care?
- How do you go about creating the right culture for an organization, team or individuals?

The Department of Trade and Industry (DTI, 1997) suggest that an effective organization recognizes that shared culture, shared learning, shared effort and shared information and shared working relationships, having

Table 6.2 Cultural factors enabling and inhibiting collaborative working

Cultural factors	Rationale
Openness and honesty	To state how you feel about a situation whether it is good or not so good. To encourage reporting of untoward incidents, exemplars of good practice and to celebrate success and learn from when things have not gone so well
Trust between employees and employers	To foster an environment where staff feel safe to whistle-blow or voice concerns without retribution
Undervaluing staff	To create a feeling of confidence and pride in one's daily role and to appreciate how the role relates to others so issues akin to boundaries are avoided
Not rewarding staff	Recognizing that innovation requires hard work and reward. Focusing on developing a framework for acknowledging, rewarding and celebrating innovation and change could avoid the development of low morale that may be regarded as an inhibitor to the provision of quality care
Stifling innovation	Fostering a working organization and culture based on reciprocity and appreciation of roles and responsibilities through shared working, learning and rewards
Lack of transparency	Encouraging and listening to opinions both internally and externally and responding to them

mutual respect for difference in professional groups/disciplines and roles and responsibilities, are the keys to high productivity and quality. For collaborative working to become a reality for any health and social care organization, the cultural factors outlined in Table 6.2 need addressing, as the rationale column suggests.

A health and social care organization that is innovative, involving staff from all levels of the organization and patients/carers, is an ideal foundation for fostering collaborative working. As advocated by Haslock (1999), to improve standards requires the development of an open, supportive learning environment and culture that focuses an educating as opposed to naming, blaming and shaming. The challenge for some health and social care organizations, teams and individuals is how to develop this culture within their respective workplace. The starting point for addressing the questions associated with culture is to establish the type of culture within your present organization or team. Hawkins and Shohet (1989) cited in Northcott (1999) identify five types of culture:

Blame – a culture that seeks to address mistakes and apportion blame to individuals

Bureaucratic – an overreliance on rules, regulations, procedures and policies at the jeopardy of individual personal judgement.

Mistrust (watch your back) – an overcompetitive environment that seeks to embarrass departments and individuals and stifles innovation, creativity and change.

Reactive (knee-jerk) – short-term management plans and dealing with the problem. No long-term vision and action plan.

Proactive (leaning) – encouraging learning and development. Learning with each other and from when things go well and not so well.

Case study 6.1 Proactive culture leading to a learning organization

It is clear from the above that a proactive culture of learning is the most suitable for fostering a working organization culture and environment that supports collaborative working. This is because an environment or culture that seeks to apportion blame only leads to secrecy, mistrust and a failure to report mistakes, with a knee-jerk reaction to resolving the incidents; for example, a health and or social care professional administers the wrong medication to a patient, which results in no harm to the patient. The immediate response of management was to discipline the member of staff, who received a written warning on their personal file – a classic case of reactive knee-jerk culture that actively seeks to apportion blame because of failure to adhere rigidly to policy and procedure. This example demonstrates the element of culture that is bureaucratic, reactionary and closed, by blaming individuals.

Alternatively, in an open learning or proactive culture the incident would have been dealt with by exploring and establishing the facts before apportioning blame, with the systems and processes reviewed before any action was taken against the individual. This approach treats the whole incident as a learning opportunity for the individual and the organization and where possible offers support, if needed, to the individual and patient concerned. The lessons learnt from the incident are disseminated throughout the organization, in an anonymous way to avoid naming, blaming and shaming of individuals, to avoid a recurrence of this type of event. It is evident that for collaborative working to succeed, an environment is necessary that is open, honest, trusting and willing to learn from its mistakes and share good practices. The preferred culture to promote this type of environment is that of a 'constructive culture', a culture that:

- promotes learning
- learns from experiences and mistakes
- communicates to all
- collaborates between all levels of the organization

- rewards, values and develops staff
- is genuinely committed to quality improvement
- values diversity and treats all as equal partners.

This type of open or transparent culture takes 'time, and requires working for collaborative results rather than relying upon domination or compromise as a quick fix' (Northcott, 1999: 10). Some health and social care organizations will require a cultural change to successfully support collaborative working. This will not be easy and will require careful management and good leadership.

Management

The management style of a health and social care organization will have a significant impact on collaborative working. Management and leadership go hand in hand but there is a difference between the two. Marquis and Hutson (2000) suggest that management is about guiding and directing staff and resources and is concerned with having the power and legitimate authority for particular tasks and duties. Essentially, management is primarily concerned with outcomes and the manipulation of resources to achieve the desired outcome(s). For example, in relation to clinical governance the chief executives of health care organizations are accountable to parliament for the implementation of the clinical governance framework, ensuring clinical quality along with meeting financial and performance targets – targets such as those outlined in the Patient's Charter (DoH, 1992): to be seen in the outpatient department within half an hour of their specified waiting time; to be seen by a consultant within 13 weeks from the time of GP referral. These are all standards that require achievement through the process of delegation to other personnel within the organization. Management in this instance is about the transferring of roles and responsibilities to a specified team or individual for achieving the specific standards or desired aims and objectives.

This collaborative and participative approach to management is the type that encourages a shared responsibility and ownership of what the organization is trying to achieve. This is an essential attribute in the development, implementation, monitoring and evaluation of collaborative working where the success of the systems and processes are strongly associated with the specific management style of the lead for that part of the service. For example, if the manager or lead clinician is autocratic and not prepared to listen to the opinions of others, this will have a detrimental effect on advancing and evaluating the quality improvement programme.

Previously in health and social care, effective management was valued more than good leadership. 'In difficult times, people need leadership as well as management' (Stewart, 1996: 3) – an approach advocated within the NHS of today in addressing the factors that have led to the introduction of collaborative working and in developing new and creative ways of implementing the key systems and processes for the sharing and delivery of services. Further information on management and the management of change is detailed in Chapter 1.

Change management

Change is a complex process in which inhibitors are inherent, threatening the successful implementation of collaborative working. Utilizing a change model can help guide the change process and help to reduce obstacles that may be encountered. As already provided in Chapter 1 there are numerous change or improvement models/frameworks available to support innovation and change in the quest for collaborative working. The challenging is finding the most suitable for your need and building effective strategies to support individual reactions to change.

Reaction to change

Most health and social care professionals find change disruptive and by merely exposing the flaws of a particular practice or presenting research findings to support the rationale for change, you will still most likely face resistance. While individuals may resist, different people will respond differently. There are four main reasons why people resist change: self-interest, misunderstanding and lack of trust, difference of the situation and low tolerance for change (Kotter and Schlesinger 1997, cited in McSherry et al., 2002a, b).

The potential varied responses by individuals to a change are vast but should not be overlooked when implementing change associated with collaborative working. Managers should try and establish the views and opinions of the organization, team and individuals about the levels of tolerance, misunderstanding and interest associated with collaborative working so that the inhibitors to change can be avoided. The combination of effective management with leadership may help this process, as is briefly explored in the next section.

Leadership

Many people confuse management and leadership. Before we can proceed we need to understand the differences and relationships between leadership and management. This was eloquently described by Field Marshall Slim, cited in Stewart (1996: 3–13):

> There is a difference between leadership and management. Leadership is of the spirit, compounded of personality and vision; its practice is an art. Management is of the mind, a matter of accurate calculation. its practice is a science. Managers are necessary; leaders are essential.

As mentioned in the previous section, managers are essential for the efficiency and effectiveness of an organization and team. However, this is not to say that all good managers show the attributes that make successful leaders. For collaborative working to work, we need leaders who can 'make others feel that what they are doing matters and hence make them feel good about their work' (Stewart, 1996: 4). This notion of empowering, involving and valuing staff is fundamental in developing the culture in which collaborative working will operate effectively. Some of the essential attributes of an effective clinical leader are:

- visionary
- communicator
- facilitator
- advocator
- critical thinker
- evaluator
- respectable
- knowledgeable
- tactful.

A clinical leader will utilize these and many more essential attributes to influence and develop the organization, team and individuals. Furthermore, as outlined in Chapter 1, it is imperative to establish the types of leadership style associated with the various members of the team and how these collectively contribute to developing effective collaborations.

Communication

Communication is a recurring theme throughout all the chapters as it plays a major role in any organization's quest for excellence in practice. 'Communication seems to be about an interaction where two or more people send and receive messages, and in the process both present themselves and interpret the other' (McSherry, 1999: 198). McSherry's quotation about communication is applicable to collaborative working because, 'without clear communication, it is impossible to give care effectively, make decisions with clients and families, protect clients from threats to well-being, coordinate and manage client care, assist the client in rehabilitation, offer comfort, or teach' (Potter and Perry, 1993: 24). Effective communication is an integral ingredient for collaborative working. It is of paramount importance in ensuring effective communications between and within:

- the various systems and processes associated with the collaboration
- individual health and social care professionals both clinical and non-clinical
- organizations such as Primary Care Trusts, Strategic Health Authorities, Acute Trusts, Care Quality Commission, to name but a few.

A failure in communication between or within these organizations, teams or individuals could result in complaints about health and social care that are in the main linked to a failure in communications associated with 'staff attitudes, poor inter-team communication or lack of information for patients' (O'Neill, 2000: 817). For the systems and processes associated collaborative working to work in harmony, it is vital to have a culture that encourages open channels of communication between and within all levels of the organization, teams and individuals. Failures to actively encourage honesty, openness and 'freedom of speech' contradict the philosophy behind collaboration and the promotion of an environment where clinical excellence will flourish. 'Whistle-blowing' and the reporting of poor practices, performance or competences associated with the systems, processes or individuals should be encouraged via open two-way channels of communication between all levels of the organization.

Communication can be enhanced and improved in the clinical environment by:

- sharing of goals
- information
- learning
- roles and responsibilities.

In this way a culture based on teamwork, partnerships and mutual collaboration becomes the norm. Collaborative working is not designed to work in a unidisciplinary manner; it needs teams and the individuals within the teams to collaborate, reliant on the efficiency and effectiveness of the communications processes.

Health and social care collaboration is team-based relying on the 'direct or indirect support and influences of others, either from their own or other professions or work groups' (Northcott, 1999: 10). This point is highlighted by the NHS Circular 1999/065 where multidisciplinary and multi-agency collaboration is viewed as an essential component for improving the efficiency and effectiveness of health and social care services. Effective teamworking and multidisciplinary or multi-agency approaches to care delivery are only truly effective where communication is continuous and seamless. For example, it would be fair to state that a patient's recovery from stroke is interdependent on multidisciplinary collaboration and effective communications, not individual practices. For collaborative working to function efficiently, and effectively, health and social care professions need to have the ability to coordinate patient/carers' care by passing information to and from within the multidisciplinary team, a skill that requires effective management and leadership qualities.

If we find it difficult to communicate effectively with each other and with patients, what can one expect to find when it comes to reviewing standards and when faced with the challenge of fostering collaboration within and between organization, team or individual practices? For collaborative working to succeed, it becomes evident that communication is of paramount importance as it is the unifying factor that crosses through all team members.

To achieve effective communications in supporting collaborative working, the organization, teams and individuals need to be adequately informed. The latter can only be achieved by offering the appropriate education and training.

Education and training

The education and training needs of health and social care professionals should be considered on a wide basis to inform and educate staff within all levels of the organization about what collaborative working means, involves and associated systems and processes required for success. The education and training of staff should be based on a 'need to know basis' where the appropriate information is provided about collaborative working and how this affects them and their role. To ensure that this happens, the employee and employer have a mutual responsibility to ensure that education and training are provided at a local level. The employee should make it known, through their individual personal development plans, that they have a development need associated with collaborative working. The employer should seek to establish the educational needs of their employees, perhaps through the development and implementation of a staff 'collaborative working awareness questionnaire'. Likewise, local universities providing health and social care courses need to develop collaborative working modules to educate both their pre and post-registration health and social care students about collaborative working. The education and training programme(s) should be designed to best suit the target audience. It is imperative that all levels of the health and social care teams are aware of their educational responsibilities in informing and educating their staff about the what, why and how of collaborative working. The most important but sometimes difficult aspect in the education and training of collaborative working is in linking it to the organization, teams and individuals and in releasing personnel from their daily clinical duties to attend educational courses and so on (Phipps, 2000).

Informing the organization, team and individuals of collaborative working

The education and training needs of staff could be provided at three levels within a local health and social care organization where the information about collaborative working is designed with a specific targeted audience in mind. For example: at an organizational level all new employees of the Trust would attend the induction programme where a brief presentation on collaborative working would be given, associated with an overview of the structures and processes linked to its cause. At a team/directorate level, a specific education and training programme could be delivered via the 'rolling development programmes' where collaborative working is aligned to the specific activities of the team. Case studies, critical reflections and reviews of complaints are used as examples of where collaboration fits in with practice, accompanied by networking and sharing good and not so good practices within the teams and organizations and where necessary externally to other organizations. At an individual level, the education and training needs of the individual should be associated with learning needs established after the performance review, forming the basis of the personal development plan. These could be attendance on courses, seminars or workshops. The inhibitors for some organizations, teams and individuals is in establishing what they need to know; that is, where collaborative working relates to them and their practice and in accessing the information on collaborative working. This is where having a knowledge and understanding of collaborative working is essential if it is to become an integral part of health and social care professions' daily practice and not seen to be another obstacle to practice.

Knowledge

To ensure that all health and social care staff have sufficient knowledge and understanding of collaborative working, the education and training should be targeted to specific audiences with relevant aims and objectives that relate to and reflect the realities of their clinical or non-clinical practice. All employees should be made aware of the idea that for collaborative working to become a reality, it is everybody's business. To make certain that collaborative working becomes known and owned by all staff, educational and training programmes need to be directed to the appropriate audiences. The educational programmes on collaborative working need to cover the key components such as what is collaborative working, why is collaborative working essential for integrated teams, what are the enabling and inhibiting factors of collaborative working and how do you establish the effectiveness of collaborative working? Relevant examples and case studies are taken from real-life situations to reinforce understanding and the relevance of clinical practice to their own practice.

The development of any educational programme for teams or individuals should be linked to demands of the local organization or educational requirement highlighted via the workforce educational confederations (previously known as educational consortia). Any devised educational programmes should be:

- multi-professional
- collaborative in nature
- practically focused
- evidence-based
- utilizing a variety of teaching and learning methods
- competence-based
- evaluated regularly.

All collaborative working educational programmes should be about learning from the practical experience gained in the workplace, with the learning shared and disseminated across multi-professional boundaries. This approach to shared and problem-based learning is more likely to be successful, an approach advocated by the following statements:

> Learning in teams, developing multidisciplinary education and training across different agencies, is the way forward for creating learning environments. It will encourage healthcare professionals to work in partnerships in sharing ideas and solving problems that focus on what is important for patients (Squire, 2000: 1015).

> New approaches to undergraduate medical education, such as the introduction of problem based learning, joint education with other professional disciplines, should in time improve teamworking skills; the importance of team working has been emphasised by the General Medical Council (Scally and Donaldson, 1998: 65).

To foster this new approach to shared learning and problem-solving relating to the development, implementation, monitoring and evaluation of collaborative working of health and social care organizations, teams and individuals need to be supported.

Support

The success of collaborative working will depend on the support and resources given within the various levels of the health and social care sectors to implement such a huge innovation. Supporting infrastructures for successful collaborative working depend on collaboration, partnerships and adequate levels of resourcing at organizational, team and individual level. The support is not just about financial backing but the physical releasing or 'freeing up' of staff to develop their knowledge, understanding, skills and competence to deliver the collaborative agenda at a local or individual level. Local support for staff could be in the form of:

Clinical supervision: offering a framework for staff to identify and explore issues about the quality of care delivered, along with the identification of education and training needs in enabling them to improve their clinical competence.

Reflective practice and critical incident analysis: to help identify and resolve clinical concerns and share good practice.

Lifelong learning: the need to ensure that staff have the support to continuously develop professionally.

Performance management review: to offer support and advice in the organization's drive for continuous quality improvement.

Clinical audit: to support staff in the evaluation of care associated with set standards and guidelines.

Offering the opportunity for networking and collaboration: to encourage staff to share and learn from each other.
Professional self-regulation: offering support and encouragement for the development of the professions' and individuals' performances.

Without adequate resources and support for staff at an organization, staff team and individual level to introduce collaborative working, collaborative working will not happen. Perhaps this accounts for the government's section in the National Plan in 2000 about the 'NHS will support and value its staff' (DoH, 2000: 4), directed towards resolving the fundamental inhibitors associated with the provision of support.

Conclusion

This chapter shows how collaborative working depends on resolving the potential inhibitors that exist within the organization, teams and individuals inhibitors which, if left unresolved, will make the linking of the systems

and processes associated with the collaborative working difficult to achieve. The enablers and inhibitors can be classified into key themes associated with culture, management, leadership, communication, education and training, knowledge and support. As individual health and social care professionals, it is imperative that we understand the existence of these inhibitors and develop strategies to overcome them. Failure to embrace this challenge will make collaborative working difficult to implement in our daily practices.

Key points

- The factors influencing collaborative working can be classified as internal and external factors attributed to individuals or organizations.
- These factors can be themed into seven key headings for which strategies require development in resolving their impact at an organization, team and individual level: culture, management, leadership, communication, education and training, knowledge and support.
- Management, leadership styles and culture are three enablers and inhibitors that cannot be overlooked from either an organization, team or individual level when considering the implementation of clinical governance.
- A closer inspection of the enabling and inhibiting factors will offer positive and constructive ways of achieving clinical governance.
- Adequate support is necessary.
- Education and training for staff on clinical governance is essential.

Further reading

Allen, A. (1993) Changing theory in nursing practice, *Senior Nurse*, 13(1): 43–4.

Cullen, R., Nichols, S. and Halligan, A. (2000) NHS support team: reviewing a service – discovering the unwritten rules, *British Journal of Clinical Governance*, 5(4): 233–9.

Department of Health (DoH) (2001) *Assuring the Quality of Medical Practice: Implementing Supporting Doctors Protecting Patients*. London: DoH.

Department of Health (DoH) (2001a) *Interim Guidance on Post-mortem Examinations*. Available online at www.doh.gov.uk/postmortem.htm (accessed 5 January 2010).

Department of Health (DoH) (2001b) *Assuring the Quality of Medical Practice: Implementing Supporting Doctors Protecting Patients*. London: DoH.

Harvey, G. (1998) Improving patient care, *RCN Magazine*, Autumn: 8–9.

Haslock, I. (1999) Introducing clinical governance in an acute trust, *Hospital Medicine*, 60(10): 745–7.

Lancaster, J. and Lancaster, W. (1982) *The Nurse as the Change Agent*. St. Louis: MA Mosby.

References

Callaghan, L. (2006) The use of collaboration in personal outcomes, International *Journal of Health Care Quality Assurance*, 15(5): 384–99.

Chesterman, D. (2001) Learning from research perspectives in collaborative working, *Careers Development International*, 6(7): 373–83.

Collins, W. (1987) *Collins Universal English Dictionary*. Glasgow: Readers Union Ltd.

Davies, H.T.O., Nutley, S.M. and Mannion, R. (2000) Organizational culture and quality of health care, *Quality in Health Care*, 9: 111–19.

Department of Health (DoH) (1992) *The Patient's Charter: Raising the Standard*. London: DoH.

Department of Health (DoH) (2000) *National Plan*. London: DoH.

Department of Trade and Industry (DTI) (1997) *Partnership with People*. London: DTI.

Edwards, J. and Packham, R. (1999) A model for the practical implementation of clinical governance, *Journal of Clinical Excellence*, 1(1): 13–18.

Haslock, I. (1999) Introducing clinical governance in acute trust, *Hospital Medicine*, 60(10): 745–7.

Hawkins, S. and Shohet, R. (1989) *Supervision in the Helping Professions*. Milton Keynes: Open University Press.

Hunter, D. (1996) The changing role of health care personnel in health and health care management, *Social Science and Medicine*, 43(5): 799–808.

MacDonald, A. (1996) Responding to the results of the Beverly Allitt Inquiry, *Nursing Times*, 92(2): 23–5.

Marquis, B.L. and Hutson, C.J. (2000) *Leadership Roles and Management Function in Nursing: Theory and Application*, 3rd edn. Philadelphia, PA: Lippincott, Williams & Wilkins.

McSherry, R. (1999) Supporting patients and their families, in C.C. Bassett and L. Mahin (eds) *Caring for the Seriously Ill Patient*. London: Arnold.

McMurray, R. (2006) From partition to partnership: managing collaboration within a curative framework for HHS care, *International Journal of Public Sector Management* 19(3): 238–49.

McSherry, R. and Simmons, M. (2002a) The importance of research dissemination and the barriers to implementation, in R. McSherry, M. Simmons, and P. Abbott (eds) *Evidence-informed Nursing: A Guide for Clinical Nurses*. London: Routledge.

McSherry, R. and Warr, J. (2008) *An Introduction to Excellence in Practice Development*. Maidenhead: Open University Press.

McSherry, R., Simmons, M. and Abbott, P. (2002b) *Evidence-informed Nursing: A Guide for Clinical Nurses*. London: Routledge.

National Health Service (NHS) Institute for Innovation and Improvement (2009) *The Leadership Qualities Framework*. Available online at www.executive.modern.nhs.uk/framework/deliveringtheservice/collaborativeaspx (accessed 4 February 2010).

Northcott, N. (1999) Organizational effectiveness, *Nursing Times Learning Curve*, 3(1): 10.

O'Neill, S. (2000) Clinical governance in action: part 4: communication, *Professional Nurse*, 16(1): 816–17.

Phipps, K. (2000) Nursing and clinical governance, *British Journal of Clinical Governance*, 5(2): 69–70.

Potter, A.P. and Perry G.A. (1993) *Foundations of Nursing: Concepts, Process and Practice*. London: Mosby.

Ramsey, S. (2001) Audit exposes UK's worst serial killer, *The Lancet*, 357: 123–4.

Scally, G. and Donaldson, L.J. (1998) Clinical governance and the drive for quality improvement in the new NHS in England, *British Medical Journal*, 317: 61–5.

Squire, S. (2000) Clinical governance in action: part 7: effective learning, *Professional Nurse*, 16(4): 1014–15.

Stewart, R. (1996) *Leading in the NHS: A Practical Guide*, 2nd edn. London: Macmillan Business.

Acknowledgement

The chapter has been reproduced with kind permission from Blackwell Publishing and is adapted from McSherry and Pearce (2007) Identifying and exploring the barriers to the implementation of clinical governance, in R. McSherry and P. Pearce (2007) *Clinical Governance. A Guide to Implementation for Healthcare Professionals*. Blackwell Oxford: Publishing.

PART 3
User-focused care

7 Exploring the meaning of user involvement and making it happen

Lee-Ann Fenge and Katie Tucker

Introduction

This chapter briefly outlines the background to service user/carer and lay involvement in health and social care practice development, followed by a detailed outline of the drivers for their involvement, frameworks to support their involvement, and some of the challenges to achieving this. To illustrate this, a number of activities and a case study are used. The chapter is different from Chapters 8 and 9 by exploring the meaning of user involvement and making it happen.

Background

A wide range of terms related to the involvement of users of services and carers are found within health and social care literature and policy. This has encouraged widespread debate about what such terms mean, including the use of labels such as 'patient', 'service user', 'consumer' or 'lay participant' (Deber et al., 2005; Beresford, 2005). Such labels illustrate the power divide that exists between users of services and service providers, and can have a disempowering effect in terms of preserving the status quo of 'professional' and 'non-professional'. Ultimately, this may work against the process of user involvement 'if those that it refers to and those that use it see it as stigmatizing' (Hefferman, 2006: 826). The use of certain labels can be problematic for user groups, particularly if they reinforce notions of powerlessness and passivity, such as the term 'patient' that implies passivity and acceptance of the medical model of psychiatry (Rudman, 1996). Those within the user movement try to distance themselves from psychiatry and from the attributions of being a patient. They use a variety of terms to describe themselves – consumers, service users, survivors, clients, ex-users or ex-patients (Holling, 2001). It is also important to consider that all these terms fail to recognize those that need services but cannot access them (Downe et al., 2007: 3).

A recent clarification of terms within the Social Care Institute for Excellence (SCIE) document developed in partnership with Shaping Our Lives National User Network is a useful reference point within this debate. This suggests that the term 'service user should always be based on self-identification' (SCIE, 2007: vii). It encompasses meanings associated with unequal and oppressive relationships within the state and society; with entitlement to welfare services; and a shared experience across a wide range of people who use services (SCIE, 2007: vii).

Activity 7.1 Reflective question

Write down the different terms used to describe user/carer/volunteer, etc. involvement that are used in your work environment. How might these terms either 'include' or 'exclude' individuals in practice development activities?

Read on and compare your answers with the remainder of the chapter.

Origins of user and carer involvement

Historically, society has expected service users to be accepting and grateful for whatever was offered rather than demanding better quality services (Banks, 2005). English society locates care professionals in a position of power with the innate assumption being they are best placed to make decisions about how people's needs are met. Compounding this presumption, the welfare system contains innate conceptions about the capacity of the person using the system. Even for individuals normally seen as the most competent when using the welfare system, they become adversely affected by group dynamics. Often, in fact for generations, these individuals have been infantilized and given little choice about what care services they receive (Bruder et al., 2005). Only in very recent English history have people using care services challenged the assumption that their capacity to make decisions is impaired (DoH, 2000; Rapley, 2003).

Since 1974, care professionals have expressed the intention to support people to obtain care packages, which reflect what they want and not what is available (Cassum and Gupta, 1993). Professionals and politicians expound the view that the care industry should no longer accept the concept of people being passive recipients of care (Department of Health, 2005b, 2006) and that care professionals and the industry must promote people's right to decide how their care needs are best met (Department of Health, 2005a, 2006, Netten et al., 2004, Petch et al., 2005). The discourse throughout professional and political literature has stated that people who use services need to be actively consulted about how they would like their needs met (McCormack, 2002). This represented a major shift in the professional's perception of the role of the service user.

In conjunction or probably more correctly as a forerunner to this change in care professional's perception, disability pressure groups have come to the fore (Reed and McCormack, 2005). In the late 1970s the voice of people with disabilities really started to emerge and they ardently challenged the status quo. People with disabilities have lobbied hard in political and social circles demanding that their place in society is valued (Hyde, 2000). They have raised the profile of the inequalities people experience and their right to live ordinary lives (Bruder et al., 2005). This in part was sparked by the successful challenge in the USA to the societal norm and the subsequent introduction legislation supporting the rights of people with disability. In England the various service representative groups became increasingly vocal about their rights to make decisions and be involved in the development of services (Netten et al., 2004). In response, the White Paper, *Valuing People* (DoH, 2000), promoted using person-centred practices.

Yet *Valuing People*: the White Paper, *A New Strategy for Learning Disability for the 21st Century* (DoH, 2008) found that people with learning disabilities continue to fail to be listened to and have their wishes valued. This supported the findings from the Learning Difficulties Audit (Healthcare Commission, 2007a). Thus, although much rhetoric has been heard in many respects, people with disabilities continue to be infantilized and therefore deemed unable to make even the simplest choice (Bruder et al., 2005). The reasons for this is that people with disabilities lack the opportunity to express their opinion and be in control of the way their needs are met (Sommerlad, 2004).

Care professionals hold a position of power and therefore control what resources people with disabilities are offered. Their decisions around what provisions within the welfare state are allocated is obviously contingent on availability of resources but also the values practitioners hold (Seedhouse, 2005). Values are created from learning and experience. Until recently people who use services have been predominantly excluded from contributing to the development of professionals' values. They have been seen, particularly through the medical model, as inert and passive recipients of care (Rapley, 2003).

Researchers and practitioners recognized that to engender the change to a person-centred practice it had to involve finding out what people actually wanted; that in order to achieve this goal, people with disability and carers needed to become full participants in the development of policy and services (Petch et al., 2005). This shift in cultural expectation is leading to changes in the way practitioners work (Carpenter, 1997). Practitioners are being equipped with the tools to measure care services' success at tailoring provision so it meets the wishes of the service user (Netten et al., 2004). Also participative work is being conducted across the health and social care sector, with the development of patient experts, people with disabilities sitting on local partnership boards actively shaping services in local authorities and general consultation (Innes et al., 2006). Plus care regulators involve people using care services in reference groups designing assessment frameworks, visiting and assessing service provision and in the managerial boards (CSCI, 2008).

Drivers for users and user involvement

The White Paper, *Our Health, Our Care, Our Say* (DoH, 2006), clearly sets the mandate for change. Throughout this White Paper people who use health and social care services were portrayed as competent, able individuals who were more than capable of making informed decisions.

> People say they want services that help them realise their potential and make the most of their life chances. Services that offer them real choices about the care they use, flexible services that respect and fit with their lives; fair and non discriminatory services and the chances to have the same opportunities and to take the same risks as anyone else (CSCI, 2007a).

This position has given direction for many political and governmental drivers and the jargon used to describe this is personalization. In 2008 a local authority circular was issued entitled 'Putting People First' and this ratcheted up the requirement to make sure services were developed with the individual and reflected their aspirations.

However, the welfare system contains innate conceptions of the person using the system and their capacity. Even for individuals normally seen as the most competent, their abilities and competence is often questioned once they are using welfare systems. Power differentials and group dynamics can readily be seen at play in the welfare system. The professionals, being the 'in-group', perceive themselves as more able, more competent and of more value than the 'other-group', the service users (Miell and Dallos, 1996). Stiggelbout et al. (2004) described six moral concepts of interaction, which encapsulates these dynamics (Table 7.1). The six constructs they present outline the service user and how their level of assured autonomy is interwoven with care professionals' belief systems.

Table 7.1 illustrates that in terms of the lived experience of service users, the people working with them will use all six concepts at various times. It is important to highlight, as indicated by the star rating, that all concepts are highly relevant when service users are to be engaged with innovation, change and evaluation of care/services. Furthermore, these stars will to various extents impact the level of involvement services users and carers have when developing services. Publications such as *A Life Like No Other: A National Audit of Services for People with Learning Difficulties* (Healthcare Commission, 2007a), The Mansell Report (Mansell, 2007), *Valuing People* (DoH, 2008) and the report on *Commissioning Services for People with Learning Disabilities and Complex Needs* (CSCI et al., 2009) have all found that people's choices and wishes at best are offered lip service. Although the good intention is to actively involve people who use services in the development and evaluation of services, this does not happen. Therefore, it can be concluded that there are conflicting drivers; some in favour of involvement and empowerment yet others working against this (Bromell and Hyland, 2007).

Table 7.1 Six moral concepts of interaction and relevance to user involvement

Construct	Meaning	Relevance to user involvement engagement
• **Liberal legal concepts of freedom**	Presents the service user as requiring protection from the unwanted interference of others. This principle is directed at the carers and infers the service user is a passive recipient of care	*****
• **The liberalist individualist concept of autonomy**	Presents the service user who can actively choose and decide what type of care they need. The service user is seen as able to understand the information they are presented with, weigh it up and make a rational decision	*****
• **Autonomy as a critical reflection within the theory of procedural independence**	Allows scope for paternal behaviour. The service user is seen as competent and able to reflect on the information they are presented with. Because the service user has this capacity, it then becomes acceptable for them to choose to devolve their decision to the health professional; thus allowing the health and social care professionals to make the decisions about the best treatment and care options	*****
Actual autonomy	As identification refers to decisions being based on one's own values; therefore, a health care professional can make the decision for the service user as long as the professional believes that they have matched this individual's expectations	*****
Socratic autonomy	States that the vulnerability of the service user makes the concept of autonomy essentially fragile. Thus the individual is depicted as unable to make decisions. It is therefore expected that health care professionals will fulfil the role as supporter in decision-making and base their decisions on what would be in the best interest of the service user	*****
Autonomy as negotiated consent	Promotes shared decision-making. This emphasizes the need for both the service user and health care professional to have a mutual understanding of what the situation involves so any proposed actions and decisions about care can be negotiated	*****

Note: 5-star rating where no star = not relevant through to 5 star = highly relevant.

Source: Adapted from Stiggelbout et al. (2004)

Models and frameworks for user and carer involvement

As the previous sections of this chapter have suggested, issues of power and ownership are central components when involving users of services and carers in research, education and practice development. One model, which can be used to explore issues of power within such processes, is offered by Whitmore and McGee (2001). This model identifies six principles for working with disempowered groups by exploring issues of participation and empowerment. This encourages professionals interested in developing practice alongside users of services to focus on issues of equality and ownership throughout the process.

> 1 Non-intrusive collaboration – including ownership of the project by the group.
> 2 Mutual trust and genuine respect.
> 3 Solidarity – all humanity is connected by a common journey and shared destiny.
> 4 Mutuality and equality – everyone's interests are important.
> 5 A focus on process – informal interaction that goes beyond a detached working relationship, and respects others' cultures.
> 6 Language as an expression of culture and power.
>
> *Source:* (Whitmore and McGee, 2001: 396–7)

Just as there are different ways of being involved in practice development activities, there are different levels of involvement. These different levels of involvement themselves may be linked to different approaches to practice development activity. For example, Beresford (2005) suggests that user participation falls into one of two broad categories:

- *Managerialist/consumerist* – where the main goal is to modify/improve service systems with no real intention of redistributing power.
- *Democratic* – where the aim is to improve people's lives, with the ultimate goal being empowerment, whereby people are empowered to take greater control over the situation.

A useful model to review levels of participation is Arnstein's (1971: 3) ladder of citizen participation (Figure 7.1), which outlines a continuum of participation from manipulation (non-participation) to citizen control (citizen power).

This model suggests that at one end of the continuum practice may involve merely 'informing' users of services how a particular area of practice is going to change. At the other end of the continuum the change is initiated by the users of services themselves. This might be seen as a grass-roots approach to practice development. Involving users of services and carers has also been highlighted by Hanley et al. (2003) who suggests a simplified model of Arnstein's work (Figure 7.2).

8 Citizen control]
]
7 Delegated] ---------▶ Degrees of citizen power
]
6 Partnership]

5 Placation]
]
4 Consultation] ---------▶ Degrees of tokenism
]
3 Informing]

2 Therapy]
]---------▶ Non participation
1 Manipulation]

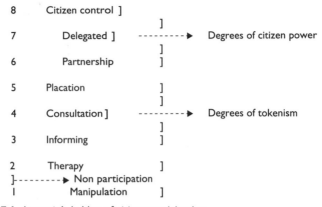

Figure 7.1 Arnstein's ladder of citizen participation

CONSULTATION ◀———▶ COLLABORATION ◀———▶ USER CONTROL

Figure 7.2 Hanley's continuum of involvement

Consultation can be seen as asking users of services and carers about their views on a particular practice development issue, and maybe at a one-off event such as a meeting whereby views are being sought on a particular policy or approach. Collaboration may be seen as a more active ongoing partnership with users of services who may join a steering group or committee, and have an ongoing involvement in the delivery of a service or project. User-controlled involvement usually signifies that the locus of power is with the users of services/carers.

Allain et al. (2006) provide an account of one university's experience of educational practice development by the involvement of users of services and carers in the delivery of the new undergraduate and postgraduate degrees using Arnstein's ladder of empowerment. This concludes that initial involvement started at rung one (manipulation) but quickly developed to rung four (consultation) and then to rung five (placation) (Allain et al. 2006: 412). Involvement is therefore an organic process, which develops and grows within a supportive partnership.

Activity 7.2 Reflective question

Think of your own practice context and where it sits in terms of Arnstein's ladder of citizen participation and the involvement of users of services/carers/volunteers, and so on, in practice development activities. How might this position be improved?

Read on and compare your answers with the chapter.

Why user and carer involvement is important in achieving excellence in practice

A range of evidence suggests that user and carer involvement in all aspects of practice development, including the education of professionals, research and service development initiatives, has benefits for all those involved (Carr, 2004; GSCC, 2004; Levin, 2004). These processes recognize the expertise of non-professionals, enabling them to share their own experiences as recipients of practice and service provision. This assists practitioners to appreciate that there are multiple realities that exist in everyday practice (Westhues et al., 2008), and as a result challenges the traditional academically defined knowledge base of practice. Practice therefore becomes enriched through the lived experiences of users of services and carers (Glasby and Beresford, 2006), resulting in practice development that responds not only to professional interests but also to the needs and aspirations of those that use and benefit from service provision.

Case study 7.1 Examples of user/carer/lay participant involvement

The Gay and Grey project provides one example of practice development involving users of services and volunteers. This was funded for three years by the Big Lottery Fund, and was a joint initiative between Help and Care, a voluntary agency working with older people in Dorset, and Bournemouth University. This project was among the very first in the UK to undertake participative action research with older lesbians and gay men. A core group of up to 20 volunteers were involved in the project, and they were self-identified non-heterosexuals (lesbians and gay men), aged between 55 and 85 years. It aimed to support and facilitate older lesbians and gay men to engage in research about their experiences of social exclusion and marginalization. It was anticipated that the findings from the project would help to inform practice development initiatives for local health and social care providers, but the project also involved volunteers in elements of practice development themselves.

Source: Gay and Grey (2006)

Two of the broad aims of the project were to:

1 identify the factors and issues that contribute to older lesbian and gay men's exclusion from the wider community of older people, the gay community itself and from the support, services and activities available for older people
2 identify how these issues could be addressed and consequently promote greater social inclusion.

This project took place against a backdrop of an increasing emphasis on working in partnership with older people (*Older People – Independence and Well Being*, Audit Commission, 2004), and a need for health and social care practice development to demonstrate greater interaction and partnership with older lesbians and gay men 'to reflect truly both anti-oppressive practice and the value of diversity' (Pugh, 2005: 217).

The project demonstrated that the involvement of volunteers in ways that are other than tokenistic requires commitment and time, so that mutual trust and respect can develop (Fenge, 2008). However, the Gay and Grey project does demonstrate how marginalized groups can have a central role in developing practice through dialogue and joint working.

In a joint project carried out by CSCI et al. (2009), people with learning disabilities and family carers were an integral part of the development of an assessment framework and subsequent review of several areas commissioning practice. The project team were mandated to develop a means to assess how successful commissioning departments in both councils and Primary Care Trusts were at making sure that services were provide for people with learning disabilities and complex needs. This assessment was not purely to look at whether people received appropriate services but were actively involved in making sure these meet their needs.

The team felt it was essential to actively involve people with learning disabilities and family carers from the offset (CSCI, 2006). Therefore, 10 people with learning disabilities and 6 carers from various organizations such as the National Forum formed part of a reference group. They, along with the other members such as representatives from the SCIE and the Department of Health, shaped the whole project. The reference group comprised of 25 people in total. This group were integral to the development of the Assessment Framework and reviewing the project methodology.

Then during the actual review of the area's commissioning practices people with learning disabilities also became paid members of the review teams. Each review team consisted of a CSCI service inspector, Healthcare Commission assessor, Mental Health Act Commissioner, person with learning disabilities and their supporter, family carer and a valuing people commissioner. They visited a local authority area, different team members spent a day with five people who used various types of services, held open sessions and interviewed care managers, commissioning and senior staff in councils and PCTs. In addition, people with learning disabilities completed mystery shopping such as going to a local GP practice, hospital or social services department to see how easy it was to get information (CSCI et al., 2009).

The project found that involving people with learning disabilities and carers in this way proved to be invaluable. The insights they offered were about what was important in both the assessment framework and the way the reviews were conducted (CSCI et al., 2009). In line with previous projects of a similar nature, the inclusion of people with an implicit understanding of individuals' lived experience rather than merely trying to walk in their shoes ensured the right questions were asked (Healthcare Commission, 2007b). However, it also highlighted that care professionals still remained tied to some hierarchical value base and found it difficult to listen to what people were saying. But innate cultural assumptions do take time to change (Delanty, 1997).

Challenges to user involvement

There are many barriers to the meaningful inclusion of users of services and carers in practice development initiatives and service planning. As discussed in the previous section, involvement in ways that are other than tokenistic require commitment and time. Time is needed to build up trust and interpersonal relationships, to negotiate aims and responsibilities, and to ensure that all concerned possess skills needed for the task. In a study of organizations in a process of change to more user involvement models of working, Robson et al. (2003) found the following barriers:

- fragmentation rather than a whole organization approach
- glass ceilings
- initiatives that are more about image than a belief in user involvement
- staff turnover.

Working in partnership with users of services and carers does not guarantee an approach that will empower all those involved. As mentioned previously, the very terms used to identify user involvement such as 'service user' and 'carer' can be stigmatizing and excluding (Hefferman, 2006). Using participatory approaches in research and practice development may be perceived to be empowering but this may 'disguise or minimize other axes of difference' (Gavanta and Cornwall, 2001: 75). Individuals may be drawn into particular projects or development activities because they share a feeling of solidarity with each other. However, other minority voices can be excluded through such processes, and as a result become silenced (Fenge, 2008).

A key issue here is the 'representativeness' of those users and carers that become involved. The nature of group processes within user involvement groups can lead to what Lennie (2005) describes as 'political disempowerment', where certain participants take control of particular aspects of the project and agenda. As a result some users and carers may perceive that their needs are not accommodated within particular projects or organizations, and if they then leave the group it is possible that 'untold truths' may occur (Lundy and McGovern, 2006). Beresford (2007) warns that unless diversity in user involvement is addressed, then it may in fact reinforce rather displace existing exclusion and marginalization of certain groups. For example, questions concerning the representativeness of the user groups involved in social work education have led some lecturers to question its value. Users and carers contribute views based on their own experience, which may or may not be typical. Felton and Stickley's (2004) findings suggest that some lecturers feel that service users should be 'representative' to be of value.

One way to promote an emancipatory approach to practice development with community groups, users of services and carers is through developing community-university or community-organizational partnerships (Savan, 2004). Institutional barriers to this approach have been identified by Savan (2004: 380) and Suarez-Balcazar et al. (2005: 96), which highlight the following:

- Extra resources are required to develop and maintain such partnerships.
- The emphasis in academia on theoretical work and publications can undermine interest in applied research and practice development with policy outcomes.
- Lack of funding for applied community-based research and practice development activities relative to more traditional scholarly activity.
- Conflicts of interest.
- Time commitment.

A major barrier to involvement is the payment of users and carers. The principle of paying users of services for their time and expenses is an accepted aspect of involvement (Levin, 2004: 25). However, a report by the CSCI (2007b) suggests that a major barrier to involvement of users is the current benefit system. Four main barriers were identified:

1 Most people on benefits are limited to earnings of £5, £10 or £20 a week.
2 People fear being wrongly disallowed incapacity benefit.
3 Reimbursed expenses (for travel, personal assistants and replacement carers) can be treated as earnings.
4 Even if people offer to be involved for free, as volunteers, their benefits can be affected by the notional earning rule (CSCI, 2007b: 2)

Recommended solutions to the current benefit barriers to involvement include reforming the benefits system to ensure that payment for involvement should be treated in the same way for all types of benefits; reimbursed travel expenses should not be treated as earnings; and the notional earning rule should not be applied to involvement activity (CSCI, 2007b: 3).

Conclusion

This chapter has focused on the importance of involving users of services/carers, and so central within practice development processes. As previously discussed, excellence is an ever-changing term and difficult to define. However, it is important to remember that excellence needs to be defined by those that use and receive services. It is therefore vital that users of services and carers have a central role in informing practice development through their expertise as recipients of health and social care provision. Their lived experiences and insights can challenge both hearts and minds in practice contexts.

The challenge for health and social care practice is to develop, implement and evaluate models and systems, support the active engagement of users of services and carers, and avoid tokenism or the marginalization of such perspectives.

Key points

- There is a need for health and social care organizations to address and respond to the growing policy aimed at valuing the 'expertise' of users of services/patients/carers. Health care policy and legislation has confirmed this principle as a central tenet of the modernization agenda.
- Working in partnership with users of services/patients/carers can be seen to operate on a continuum, from low level involvement through consultative processes through to user-driven developments at the other end of the continuum.
- Despite the potential benefits of involving users of services/patients/carers in practice development, it is imperative that individuals, teams and organizations understand that adopting participative approaches can sometimes mean that certain disadvantaged groups become further silenced by political disempowerment.
- Working in partnership with users of services/patients/carers demands trust, time commitment and funding. In practice these issues can prove challenging, particularly issues associated with payments.
- To work effectively and collaboratively with people who use services care, professionals need to spend time reflexively understanding their innate value base and how this impacts on their behaviour.

Further reading

Beresford, P. (2000) User's knowledge and social work theory, *British Journal of Social Work*, 30: 489–503.

Department of Health (DoH) (2007) *Putting People First: A Shared Vision and Commitment to the Transformation of Social Care*. London: Her Majesty's Stationery Office (HMSO).

Fink, J. (ed.). (2004) *Care: Personal Lives and Social Policy*. Milton Keynes: Open University Press.

Harris, J., Foster, M., Jackson, K. and Morgan, H. (2005) *Outcomes for Disabled Service Users*. University of Kent: Social Policy Research Unit.

Hutton, J. (2006) *Active Welfare State: Matching Rights with Responsibility*. London: Department for Work and Pensions.

Useful links

Care Services Improvement Partnership www.csip.org.uk
In Control www.in-control.org.uk
Care Services Improvement Partnership Valuing People Support Team
www.valuingpeople.gov.uk
CSIP Networks www.networks.csip.org.uk

References

Allain, L., Cosis Brown, H., Danso, C., et al. (2006) User and care involvement in social work education – a university case study: manipulation or citizen control? *Social Work Education*, 25(4): 403–13.

Arnstein, S.R. (1971) A ladder of citizen participation, *Journal of the Royal Town Planning Institute*, April: 1–6.

Audit Commission (2004) *Older People – Independence and Wellbeing: The Challenge for Public Services*, London: Audit Commission Publications.

Banks, P. (2005) New hurdles for integrated commissioning? *Journal of Integrated Care*, 13: 21–6.

Beresford, P. (2005) Theory and practice of user involvement in research: making the connection with public policy and practice, in L. Lowes and I. Hulatt (eds) *Involving Service Users in Health and Social Care Research*. London: Routledge, pp. 6–12.

Bromell, D. and Hyland, M. (2007) *Social Inclusion and Participation: A Guide for Policy and Planning*. New Zealand Ministry of Health: Social Inclusion Policy Group.

Bruder, C., Kroese, B.S. and Bland, S. (2005) The impact of a vulnerable adult protection policy on the psychological and emotional well-being of adults with a learning disability, *The Journal of Adult Protection*, 7: 6–13.

Carpenter, J. (1997) *Choice, Information and Dignity: Involving Users and Carers in Care Management*. Bristol Policy Press: Community Care into Practice.

Carr, S. (2004) *Has Service User Participation Made a Difference to Social Care Services?* London: Social Care Institute for Excellence (SCIE).

Cassum, E. and Gupta, H. (1993) *Quality Assurance for Social Care: A Practical Guide*. London: Longman.

Commission for Social Care Inspection (CSCI) (2006) *Real Voices, Real Choices*. London: Department of Health (DoH).

Commission for Social Care Inspection (CSCI) (2007a) *State of Social Care*. London: Department of Health (DoH).

Commission for Social Care Inspection (2007b) *Benefit Barriers to Involvement: Finding Solutions*. London: Department of Health (DoH).

Commission for Social Care Inspection (CSCI) (2008) *Raising Voices: Views on Safeguarding Adults*. London: Department of Health (DoH).

Commission for Social Care Inspection (CSCI), Healthcare Commission and Mental Health Act Commission (2009) *Commissioning Services for People with Learning Disabilities and Complex Needs*. London: Department of Health (DoH).

Deber, R., Kraetschmer, N., Urowitz, S. and Sharpe, N. (2005) Patient, consumer, client, or customer: what do people want to be called? *Health Expectations*, 8: 345–51.

Delanty, G. (1997) *Social Science: Beyond Constructivism and Realism*. Milton Keynes: Open University Press.

Department of Health (DoH) (1999) *Patient and Public Involvement in the New NHS*. London: Her Majesty's Stationery Office (HMSO).

Department of Health (DoH) (2000) *Valuing People*. London: Her Majesty's Stationery Office (HMSO).

Department of Health (DoH) (2001) *The Expert Patient: A New Approach to Chronic Disease Management for the 21st Century*. London: Her Majesty's Stationery Office (HMSO).

Department of Health (DoH) (2002) *Requirements for Social Work Training*. London: Her Majesty's Stationery Office (HMSO).

Department of Health (DoH) (2005a) *Putting People in Control of their Care*. London: NOVAS.

Department of Health (DoH) (2005b) *Independence, Choice and Well-being*. London: Her Majesty's Stationery Office (HMSO).

Department of Health (DoH) (2006) *Our Health, Our Say, Our Say: A New Direction for Community Services*. London: Her Majesty's Stationery Office (HMSO).

Department of Health (DoH) (2008) *Valuing People: A New Strategy for Learning Disability for the 21st Century*. London: Her Majesty's Stationery Office (HMSO).

Downe, S., McKeown, M., Johnson, E., Koloczek, L., Grunwald, A. and Malihi-Shoja, L. (2007) The UCLan community engagement and service user support (Comensus) project: valuing authenticity, making space for emergence, *Health Expectations*, 10(4): 1–15.

Felton, A. and Stickley, T. (2004) Pedagogy, power and service user involvement, *Journal of Psychiatric and Mental Health Nursing*, 11: 89–98.

Fenge, L. (2008) Striving towards inclusive research: an example of participatory action research with older lesbians and gay men, *British Journal of Social Work*, published online, 6 November

Gavanta, J. and Cornwall, A. (2001) Power and knowledge, in P. Reason and H. Bradbury (eds) *Handbook of Action Research: Participative Inquiry and Practice*. London: Sage Publications.

Gay and Grey in Dorset (2006) *Lifting the Lid on Sexuality and Ageing*. Dorset: Help and Care Development Ltd.

General Social Care Council (GSCC) and Social Care Institute for Excellence (SCIE) (2004) *Living and Learning Together: Conference Report*. London: GSCC SCIE.

Glasby, J. and Beresford, P. (2006) Who knows best? Evidenced-based practice and the service user contribution, *Critical Social Policy*, 26(1): 268–84.

Hanley, B., Bradburn, J., Barnes, M., Evans, C. and Goodare, H. (2003) *Involving the Public in NHS, Public Health and Social Care Research: Briefing Notes for Researchers*, 2nd edn. London: Involve.

Healthcare Commission (2007a) *A Life Like No Other: A National Audit of Services for People with Learning Difficulties*. London: Department of Health (DoH).

Healthcare Commission (2007b) *Report on External Evaluation of the Healthcare Commission's Audit of Services for People with Learning Difficulties*. London: Department of Health (DoH).

Hefferman, K. (2006) Does language make a difference in health and social care practice? Exploring the new language of the service user in the United Kingdom, *International Social Work*, 49: 825–30.

Holling, I. (2001) About the impossibility of a single (ex-) user and survivor of psychiatry position, *Acta Psychiatrica Scandinavica*, 104 (Suppl. 410): 102–6.

Hyde, M. (2000) From welfare to work? Social policy for disabled people of working age in the UK in the 1990s, *Disability & Society*, 15(2): 327–41.

Innes, A., McPherson, S. and McCabe, L., (2006) *Promoting Person-centred Care at the Frontline*. York: Joseph Rowntree Foundation.

Lennie, J. (2005) An evaluation capacity-building process for sustainable community IT initiatives, *Evaluation*, 11(4): 390–414.

Levin, E. (2004) *Involving Service Users and Carers in Social Work Education: Resource Guide No. 2*. London: Social Care Institute for Excellence (SCIE).

Lundy, P. and McGovern, M. (2006) Participation, truth and partiality: participatory action research, community-based truth-telling and post-conflict transition in Northern Ireland, *Sociology*, 40(1): 71–88.

Mansell, J.L. (2007) *Services for People with Learning Disabilities and Challenging Behaviour or Mental Health Needs: Report of a Project Group* (revised edition). London: Department of Health (DoH).

McCormack, B. (2002) A conceptual framework for person-centred practice with older people, *International Journal of Nursing Practice*, 9(8): 202–9.

Miell, D. and Dallos, R. (1996) *Social Interaction and Personal Relationships*. London and Milton Keynes: Sage Publications in association with the Open University Press.

Netten, A., Francis, K. and Bebbington, A. (2004) *Performance and Quality: User Experience of Home Care Services*. Kent: Personal Social Sciences Research Unit (PSSRU).

Petch, A., Coole, A. and Miller, E (2005) Focusing on outcomes; their role in partnership policy and practice, *Journal of Integrated Care*, 13: 26–31.

Pugh, S. (2005) Assessing the cultural needs of older lesbians and gay men: implications for practice, *Practice*, 17(3): 207–18.

Rapley, M. (2003) *Quality of Life Research*. London: Sage Publications.

Reed, J. and McCormack, B. (2005) Editorial: the involvement of service users in care service and policy; comments and implications for nursing development, *Journal of Clinical Nursing*, 14: 41–2.

Robson, P., Begum, N. and Lock, M. (2003) *Developing User Involvement: Working Towards User-centred Practice in Voluntary Organisations*. Bristol: The Policy Press.

Rudman, M.J. (1996) User involvement in mental health nursing practice: rhetoric or reality? *Journal of Psychiatric and Mental Health Nursing*, 3: 385–90.

Savan, B. (2004) Community–University partnerships: linking research and action for sustainable community development, *Community Development Journal*, 39(4): 372–84.

Social Care Institute for Excellence (SCIE) (2007) *Developing Social Change Service Users Driving Culture Change*. London: Shaping Our Lives, National Centre for Independent Living and University of Leeds Centre for Disability Studies and SCIE.

Seedhouse, D. (2005) *Values-based Decision-making for the Caring Professions*. Chichester: Wiley.

Sommerlad, H. (2004) Some reflections on the relationship between citizenship, access to justice and the reform of legal aid, *Journal of Law and Society*, 31(3): 345–68.

Stiggelbout, A.M., Molewijk, A.C., Otten, W., Timmermans, D.R.M., van Bockel, J.H. and Kievit, J. (2004) Ideals of patient autonomy in clinical decision making: a study on the development of a scale to assess patients' and physicians' views, *Journal of Medical Ethics*, 30(3): 268–74. Available online at www.jmedethics.com.

Suarez-Balcazar, Y., Harper, G.W. and Lewis, R. (2005) An interactive and contextual model of community–university collaborations for research and action, *Health Education and Behaviour*, 32(1): 84–101.

Westhues, A., Ochocka, J., Jacobson, N. et al. (2008) Developing theory from complexity: reflections on a collaborative mixed method participatory action research study, *Qualitative Health Research*, 18(5): 701–17.

Whitmore, E. and McGee, C. (2001) Six street youth who could . . ., in P. Reason and H. Bradbury (eds) *Handbook of Action Research*. London; Thousand Oaks, CA: Sage Publications, pp. 396–402.

8 | Ethical issues pertaining to user involvement in practice development

Sabi Redwood

Introduction

Since 2000 there has been a social and political shift from a top-down approach of service provision in health and social care, typically led by professionals and government agencies, towards greater participation based on the experience of those receiving services. It is of course true to say that service users have previously been involved in service evaluations, but traditionally only as respondents to the questionnaires designed by clinicians or researchers. These questionnaires tend to reflect the service provider's interests and concerns, and may or may not consider the priorities of service users (Kotecha et al., 2007). Similarly, data obtained in service evaluation surveys are analysed and reported from within the parameters established by the service provider while users of services may be reluctant to be open about their opinions out of an anxiety that this might have a negative impact on the support they receive. This chapter raises and explores a number of questions:

- What are the origins or foundations of the drive towards user involvement and how do they influence the ethics of practice development projects?
- What does a move from eliciting the perspectives of the users of services merely as respondents to involving them as active participants in the developments of genuinely user-centred services actually mean in practice?
- What are the ethical and methodological implications of such a change in direction?
- How can we develop practice and plan change and interventions that are sustainable and acknowledge workload and financial burdens?

As already highlighted in Chapter 7, the complexities involved in considering the ethics of user involvement are both conceptual and practical. It is likely that situations arise where it is not possible to neatly reconcile conflicting agendas, where negotiation and creative solutions are required and where sensitive and effective communication with others is vital. This chapter aims to guide you through the use of some ideas and strategies to ensure that practice development activities meet high ethical standards. Furthermore, it at times overlaps with Chapters 7 and 9 but the focus is primarily associated with the ethical issues pertaining to user involvement in practice development and not exploring the meaning of user involvement and making it happen or indeed developing excellent service user engagement.

Background

Under the Health and Social Care Act 2001, it is a legal duty for organizations in health and social care to involve users of services and the public in the planning, monitoring and development of services. User involvement in health and social care is a central tenet of health and social care policy as is evidence-based care. However, as Harrison et al. (2002) remind us, these two elements of contemporary policy may be in tension. This tension has been borne out in a number of instances where groups of patients have requested the use of a particular treatment for which there has not been the required evidence base to be freely available. Conversely, although there may be evidence that a particular treatment is effective, it may not be acceptable to patients or meet their preferences. This tension is exacerbated by the lack of evidence that the involvement of service users leads to – or at least contributes to – positive clinical or social outcomes for individual service users (Crawford et al., 2002; Haigh, 2008).

It is important that user involvement is not seen as an entity whose existence and definition can be taken for granted. There is a need for a better understanding about how the policy of user involvement is interpreted in public service organizations and how these interpretations shape how user involvement is put into practice. Furthermore, we need to recognize the multiple meanings assigned to it and that there are multiple forms and outputs of involvement (Fudge et al., 2008). Although user involvement shares this ambiguity with many other social concepts related to health and social care such as 'empowerment' or 'quality of life' for example, as practitioners in practice development we have a responsibility to ensure that everybody involved in practice development projects and activities is clear about the purpose of their role and participation.

There are two contrasting philosophical positions (Mosquera et al., 2001) that roughly correspond to two ethical and political approaches towards user involvement; this is discussed in the following section (Table 8.1). On the one hand, user involvement can be conceived as a 'means to an end'. As such it is essentially target-oriented with the aim of containing costs and promoting efficiency and best practice. Peoples' role is not actively to participate in identifying problems or designing services or projects, but they are expected to serve the purposes of service providers. Involving service users is not intended to devolve power, but to legitimize the decisions of policy makers and service providers (Crawford et al., 2002). Conversely, user involvement can be viewed as an 'end in itself' where it is valued irrespective of tangible outcomes. It is a social process designed to enable people to identify their needs and make decisions in order to establish ways in which they can meet them.

Table 8.1 Types of user involvement in health and social care

	Service user involvement as 'means to an end'	Service user involvement as 'end in itself'
Model	Consumerist	Democratic citizenship Social and political change movements
Approach	Top-down	Bottom-up
Power to make decisions	Not devolved to service users	Partly devolved to service users
Methods	Patient/user satisfaction surveys Suggestion boxes Consultation exercises	Methods developed by service users
Underpinning values	Improvement through consumer choice Promotion of market economy Efficiency and effectiveness	Independence Autonomy Inclusion and Human rights

The attitude of professionals in health and social care to the involvement of users is also ambiguous. While there is wide agreement about the importance of the involvement of users of services in decisions about their own care or treatment options, their participation at a strategic level of service improvements and developments is more controversial. A study by Daykin et al. (2002) suggests that involvement activity is often indirect rather than direct and employs strategies such as information and feedback-gathering from users of service, patient and user satisfaction surveys, suggestion boxes or consultation exercises. It is doubtful that such methods contribute to equalizing power relationships between professionals and the users of services because professionals remain firmly in control over the information that is gathered and used to shape any outcome or change. Professionals and service providers remain the final arbiter of how much weight is attached to patients' views. Indeed, Daykin et al. (2002) report that service users were often unaware that they have been 'involved' at all and that their views were supposed to have been central. On the other hand, there were positive outcomes for users of services insofar as communication with professionals was improved even after indirect development activities. They also identify as a potential barrier to direct user involvement the duty placed on professionals in health and social care to protect service users from harm. Certain users of services are constructed as vulnerable and there is an emphasis on protection rather than on empowerment. Furthermore, despite an explicit policy drive to user involvement, there is a lack of structure within which user involvement can take place, as Evans et al. (2003: 337) point out:

> If the government is to achieve its wider aim of increasing public participation in strategic health care planning, there will need to be much greater awareness on the part of patients, the wider public and health care

professionals as to how user involvement works and the development of more accessible systems within which it can occur.

The Department of Health has identified this shortcoming and provided practical guidance for the development of local structures and cultures to promote user and public involvement (DoH, 2007, 2008a). However, as Crawford et al. (2002) point out providers may increasingly be required to demonstrate that they involve service users at more strategic levels, but they will also continue to be accountable for the decisions they make. This will create tensions for practitioners who may be working towards a more demo-cratic and empowering model of user involvement in practice development, but find it difficult to achieve without structures that devolve the power to make decisions and allocate resources. So, despite official commitment, practitioners are often unclear about exactly how to involve service users about methods to engage so-called 'hard to reach' groups and how to address the tensions that the involvement of users in practice development invari-ably produces. Programmes of education and training workshops regarding these issues are becoming available, but in order to understand fully the ethical and political implications of user involvement, it is important to move beyond the immediate practical issues and critically explore the wider implications.

Ethical implications of different approaches to user involvement

When considering the ethical aspects of user involvement, we need to be clear about the purpose of such an involvement and what it is we are trying to achieve. Is the focus of user involvement primarily concerned with eco-nomic considerations and the more effective use of resources in the provision of services? Such a focus employs the discourse of the market economy. Terms such as quality assurance and control, rights to seek redress when things have gone wrong, customer care, patient satisfaction surveys, marketing, consumer choice and consumer demand have become part of everyday vocabulary in health and social care. The empowerment of users through their involve-ment is framed in terms of enabling them to choose between services. Thus, service users are placed in the position of consumers who can decide what service to 'buy' with an expectation that such an approach will drive positive change through choice and promote the market in health and social care. Their views may also be sought in the design of services to improve efficiency and effectiveness. However, we need to be mindful that this consumerist approach is less concerned with the redistribution of power than with eco-nomics. This is in contrast to the following position supporting user involve-ment with an emphasis on participatory democracy and citizenship. Here the focus is on encouraging a bottom-up approach that is responsive to indi-vidual and community needs. The empowerment of users is framed in terms of participation in political decision-making to ensure that their interests are served. It is concerned with enabling people to have a greater say in organizations and agencies that impact on them and to exert more control over their own lives (Beresford, 2002). The values espoused are those of independence, autonomy, inclusion and human rights. A third version of user involvement, closely related to the previous one, is the movement of proactive social action (Harrison et al., 2002). It is similar to the notion of participatory democracy and citizenship, but it emphasizes the role of political, social and collective action. Here empowerment is about active campaigning for services and information not only to demand that needs and interests are met, but also to promote particular identities such as disability or homosexuality, for example.

What these positions have in common is an emphasis on users' autonomy and agency in opposition to the traditional 'medical model' approach. The paternalism and overemphasis of professional authority tended to construct individuals as belonging to medical categories and as passively receiving care and treatment designed and dispensed by those with professional knowledge and authority. User involvement seeks to work in opposition to such power in order to restore and support users' own decision-making and self-determination. However, it is important to understand the differences in the positions, in particular the differences between the first and the latter approaches to user involvement. The consumerist approach does not challenge existing power relationships at a fundamental level insofar as it retains a provider-led approach to services and policy. User involvement is seen in terms of improving these services and making them more efficient. Participatory democratic and proactive social action approaches on the other hand are explicitly about the redistribution of political power. Practitioners need to consider their role in these different approaches towards participation and how the shifts in power they advocate, or not, affects our moral responsibilities towards the users of services.

⟳ Activity 8.1 Reflective question

In relation to practice development activities in which you have been involved, to what extent were service users involved? Consider whether they followed a consumerist or democratic approach to participation.

Read on and compare your answers with the rest of the chapter.

The centrality of power

The recent trend towards human rights-based health care explicitly addresses issues such as empowerment, participation and involvement (DoH and British Institute of Human Rights, 2008). This policy drive is underpinned by a commitment to human rights, accountability and non-discrimination.

However, in order to become a reality in the lives of service users, practitioners and services managers need to consider the power relations that exist between themselves and those who require their services. Otherwise, such policies will end up simply as an exercise in window dressing or a public relations exercise rather than redressing the balance of power.

Power is a key concept in discussions about relationships in health and social care. Like so many other social phenomena, it evades precise definition. More-over, attempts at theorizing about it are usually highly contentious because different understandings of the concept suggest different ways of analysing and interpreting the way society organizes itself and the way particular struc-tures of organization affects peoples' lives. In the liberal humanist tradition, power is viewed as a possession that people grasp so that an individual or group takes power from somebody else. Here, power is a repressive tool through which another person's or group's rights are violated by preventing them from doing what they want to do (Mills, 1997). Similarly, Karl Marx was concerned with economic relations and saw power as a macro structure such as the state that functioned to support industrial capitalism and which was displayed through public institutions such as the police, the law and the church (Turner, 1997).

The French philosopher, Michel Foucault, on the other hand, challenged theories that conceptualize power as coercive and repressive in character. Instead, he saw power as dispersed and diffused throughout social relations operating at local and micro levels through specific practices, thereby pro-ducing possibilities for forms of identity and behaviour as well as restricting them. He wrote (Foucault, 1980: 39): 'Power reaches into the very grain of individuals, touches their bodies and inserts itself into their actions and atti-tudes, their discourses, learning processes and everyday lives'. He understood power not as something that some people seize and exercise over others, but as dispersed throughout social relations. Thus, individuals are not just sub-jected to power; they also exercise it. He is also very critical of the idea that power is simply about preventing someone from carrying out their wishes and limiting people's freedom. Instead, he sought to address the complexity of the wide range of social practices through which power operated including ideas about discourse, knowledge and truth. Power works through disciplin-ing practices that regulate interactions; surveillance and self-surveillance, subject to some invisible scrutiny to ensure that individuals stay within norms and do not step out of line. Power, understood this way, suggests that who we are (allowed to be) and how we (are able to) live is subject to the specific regime of power and knowledge, discourses and practices that simul-taneously enable and limit our actions. Thus, we are already made into subjects because we cannot stand outside power/knowledge that shape our identities, construe us as particular individuals and produce our specific pos-sibilities for understanding and for action. For example, being defined as 'disabled' or having 'long-term health needs' may entitle individuals to cer-tain benefits and services, but at the same time they are likely to be excluded from many activities, workplaces and financial products such as insurance or pensions. Recent national and international legislation has sought to produce equality of access in line with human rights, thus addressing some of the structural inequalities. However, everyday experiences of inequalities and discrimination are unlikely to be overcome swiftly.

A view of power such as the one proposed by Foucault (1980) has a particular relevance to health and social care. Professionals and service users are traditionally positioned in particular relationships with each other as a result of how they are defined by, for example, in terms of social status and knowledge, producing certain discourses that prescribe rules for judging what is acceptable or inappropriate, what statements are true and which are false. Power is exercised through these discourses. Discourses are not just abstract statements and words, but are 'real' insofar as they have effects on us and our relationships with others. Thus, we are made into certain subjects because we cannot stand outside these discourses that prescribe what we can be, shape our identities, construe us as particular individuals and produce our specific possibilities for understanding and for action. Yet that does not mean that we are merely subjected to power, but we can critique and resist. Indeed, critique and resistance become an ethical activity, because social power relations are usually taken for granted to such an extent that they are perceived as 'natural' and not amenable to change. Practice, which undermines such an acceptance in order to open up different possibilities, and which works from the belief that the very process of participating in change and the production of knowledge about one's own context has the potential to redress power imbalance, is more likely to become an empowering practice.

Case study 8.1 Gender identity

'Trans' or transgender people are people whose sense of gender identity (their sense of being a man or a woman) does not seem to correspond to their anatomy or physical appearance. They are often ignored in our society, or are subject to harassment, discrimination and social disapproval. Summarizing their findings in about equality for trans people in UK health and social services, Whittle et al. (2007: 5) write:

When they are seeking treatment to transition, [trans people] will start a medical process which reduces every aspect of their life and, in particular, their health down to the most minimal of issues, their trans mental health. Practitioners, at every level of medicine, ignore the trans person's abilities to cope with ongoing crises that would destroy other people, their educational standing and the nature of the actual illness they are presenting with. The fact that some qualified nursing staff will insist on calling a person who has been transitioned for over 30 years in their former gender, is indicative of the level of ignorance that exists within our health services. But are they 'our' health services?

In his foreword to *Trans: A Practical Guide for the NHS* (DoH, 2008b: 5), Surinder Sharma, the National Director for Equality and Human Rights at the Department of Health, writes:

As an employer and a provider of healthcare services, the NHS should not only comply with the law, but should also aspire to be an exemplar of good practice and seek to ensure that its services reflect the needs of the whole of our society. This means that it is essential that we strive to involve and take account of trans people's needs in the design and delivery of all our services. This doesn't just apply at the time in their lives when they need support and care to undertake the immense challenge of changing their gender identity, but throughout life.

1 Bearing in mind the discussion on power in the previous section, what are the dominant discourses that position 'trans' people as outsiders?
2 Consider some ways in which trans people can be involved in the design and delivery of services.

The document *Trans: A Practical Guide for the NHS* (DoH, 2008b) will provide some useful ideas in relation to this activity.

A philosophical and ethical commitment to service user involvement in practice development fundamentally changes the power relationship between service users and service providers and requires some structural transformation with regard to accountability, decision-making and the allocation of resources. It is unlikely that practitioners will be able to effect such a transformation on their own. However, there are ways in which practitioners can meaningfully engage with service users to bring about desired changes. An important issue to bear in mind is to focus on the service users and resist the temptation to hide their diversity and view them as a homogenous group.

Some suggestions for principles to underpin the involvement of users in practice development

Researchers in health and social care have grappled with similar issues to the ones discussed above with regard to the ethical conduct of research in which the input of service users is central. They have faced similar dilemmas in relation to the nature of the involvement. Some researchers involve service users only in selected activities whereas others have facilitated them to control the entire research process depending on whether they viewed user involvement as a policy directive to be implemented, or as a democratic project, promoting the idea that the expertise and experience of service users is as valid as that of professionals. In collaboration with service users and 'survivors' of mental health services Faulkner (2004) identified a number of principles which, although identified in relation to user participation in research, are equally valid in relation to practice development: clarity and transparency, empowerment, identity, commitment to change, respect, equality and diversity, accountability and theoretical assumptions. These principles are of course linked and in many respects overlap, but a brief discussion of each will bring into focus the salient features of each and how they relate to practice development. I present them here under the headings used by Faulkner (2004), but have added considerations in relation to practice development.

Clarity and transparency

It might be self-evident to suggest that a clear and open approach towards everybody involved in a project from the start is a prerequisite for ethical conduct. However, there are a number of points worth consideration:

Motivation

It is important that everybody involved is clear about their motivation for taking part in a collaborative project. There may be a range of reasons for service users to participate, ranging from a desire for social justice and accessible and respectful services spurred on by a sense of inequity in current provision, wishing to be involved in change and having a say in what happens, to being able to meet others in a similar situation, finding out about other services, and viewing participation as part of their recovery and rehabilitation. Professionals may be carrying out a project as part of an educational programme or a personal development plan. They might be motivated by economic or by democratic concerns. The demand for clarity and transparency requires those motivations to be declared openly.

Language

Professional language is embedded in shared understandings that are not necessarily obvious to those outside the profession. Thus, it is important to be explicit about meanings and understandings rather than take it for granted that everyone is speaking the same language. So, for example, if the aim of an activity is improvement, discussions about what constitutes an improvement must be carried out at an early stage. People whose first language is not English are likely to be doubly disadvantaged so consideration needs to be given to translation.

Tensions

Nationally defined targets that are tied to resource availability may produce tensions with priorities identified by service users. Ensuring that service users are aware of this and have an understanding of how the resources are allocated is an important responsibility of practice developers in order to raise expectations beyond what is achievable within the remit of the project. Furthermore, the possible tension between user involvement and evidence-based care also needs to be acknowledged if it arises.

Producing evidence

As indicated earlier in this chapter, there is as yet little evidence to provide insight into the benefits of service user involvement for services (Haigh, 2008). This paucity of evidence regarding the benefits of user involvement for individuals and organizations place a burden of responsibility on practice developers to document and critically discuss their work. Therefore, it is vital that built into any projects or initiatives is a carefully developed evaluation plan to ensure that processes and outcomes can be documented and widely published.

Empowerment and transformation

The discussion about power earlier in this chapter indicates that this is a contentious notion and difficult to put into practice without fundamentally changing social and political structures. However, the term 'empowerment' features heavily in professional and policy discourses to demonstrate good intentions and commitments. Yet we need to be clear that methods such as satisfaction surveys, one-off consultations and information and feedback exercises are unlikely to facilitate empowerment.

The experience of illness, disability or a life lived in difficult social and economic circumstances is a kind of experiential knowledge that is beginning to be recognized as a legitimate source of knowledge for practice development, equally important as professional knowledge. Fudge et al. (2008) report that service users' own experiential knowledge is useful both in its own right, as well as for educating health professionals, for producing information for service users and for supporting others going through similar experiences. The authors also point out that service user involvement requires 'professionals and service users to reconceptualise the traditional category of patient to accommodate the notion that service users have a contribution to make to service planning and development, a transformation that was not always easily achieved' (Fudge et al., 2008: 5). It is useful to think of this transformation as a step towards empowerment through which service users are enabled to have a voice, both in their own lives and in the public arena. However, practitioners in health and social care need to bear in mind that empowerment is not something that can be given to service users, or that they need to abdicate their own power to empower others. Such a view of empowerment would spring from a view of power as a possession. As discussed earlier in this chapter, a Foucauldian view of power as a productive force and as dispersed and circulating through social relations may be more helpful. The awareness of power as a productive process is essential for practice developers in order to bring about through enabling a linking of service user experience with wider social and political discourses. Such a project is complex insofar as it requires practitioners to listen to amplify the voice of service users while being reflexive about their own position and role in relation to practice development. Restraints on time and resources, and possibly the practitioner's own enthusiasm to bring about change and improvements, may stifle attempts to work towards user empowerment.

Identity

Identity is about who one can be and how one can act. It is not so much a finished product, but rather a process about how people define themselves and relate to others. People tend to align themselves with particular groups that shape their identity and thus may be related to ethnic origin, nationality, faith or sexual orientation. Identity is often invisible to those who belong to mainstream categories that are privileged in a particular society, for example, white, male and middle class. The effect is that discussions about identity are usually about difference and about groups who are subject to negative stereotyping and stigma that result in experiences of racism, homophobia, sexism and other oppressive attitudes. Similarly, people who are coping with specific conditions such as HIV/AIDS, mental illness, physical and intellectual disabilities, facial disfigurement and obesity, for example, are also marginalized and subject to prejudice. Often marginalized people experience prejudice for more than one reason such as gay men with HIV/AIDS, black people with a mental illness, older people with facial disfigurements or homeless people who are drug-dependent.

The acknowledgement of identity and the experiences of powerlessness, low social status and discrimination is vital to any work practice developers wish to carry out in order to meaningfully contribute to changes in practice and services. Patterson et at. (2008) point out the challenges for people who are marginalized and excluded to be actively involved because they have learnt to mistrust professionals in public services. The result may be that limited numbers of service users will volunteer to participate or that the motivation of those already involved will fade if they perceive that entrenched power imbalances are perpetuated by attempts to involve them in service and practice development initiatives.

Commitment to change

Although it is desirable to bring about positive change, it may not be possible to achieve actual change in every practice development activity. However, service improvements are unlikely to be realized through single projects. Therefore, practitioners must be careful to avoid building up unrealistic expectations and promising outcomes that are unlikely to be delivered. This does not mean that there is a lack of commitment to change. Raising awareness of crucial issues through both wide and targeted dissemination of the project and any evidence that was produced through it plays a vital role in bringing about change.

Written dissemination through reports, journal papers and short pieces for appropriate magazines will be helpful in reaching a wide audience, but oral dissemination can often reach people that written dissemination cannot. Conferences may be a suitable forum although this may only reach a certain section of your desired audience. An effective way of reaching service users is to organize a local event for all stakeholders with an interest in the practice development initiative, including service users and managers. The use of photography or filming may be useful for the visual media of television and the Internet with the caveat that consent must be sought from everyone involved.

Respect

Respect is difficult to define in practical terms because it is conveyed in the way people communicate and interact with each other. Showing regard for the value of each person, honouring difference and paying close attention to people's views are important aspects of respect. In practical terms respect is shown through the language we use, avoiding sexist language and jargon, making assumptions about people's views or resorting to biases and stereotypes. Of course, all these issues may be done at an unconscious level. Practitioners engaged in user involvement must pay particular attention to their own cultural biases and develop a particular sensitivity with regard to difference and diversity in order to avoid perpetuating inequality and exclusion.

Equality and diversity

Equality and diversity are addressed in detail in Chapter 10. They are a vital part of user involvement in practice development that aims to transform the culture and context of care in a way that is inclusive and avoids oppression and discrimination.

Accountability

Professionals in health and social care are well versed in issues of responsibility and accountability. Accountability relates to a careful consideration of the consequences of one's action and is of course as important in user involvement in practice development as it is in professional practice. In practice development and professional practice there are risks that tensions emerge between one's professional responsibilities and users' own wish to participate. Practice developers may have concerns about service users' capacity to take part in certain activities and feel it is their duty to protect service users from harm. This may be particularly applicable in mental health and palliative care settings. It is important to consider that by labelling people as 'vulnerable', we do not remove their right to self-determination.

A patronizing attitude and a belief that people are unable to cope with distress can be disabling and lead to the exclusion of the views of an important constituency.

Concepts and theories

As discussed earlier in this chapter, power relations are often rooted in assumptions, and some of these assumptions have their origins in particular models or theories. Often these assumptions are so embedded in our consciousness that they reach the status of so-called 'common sense'. Yet they are only common to those who use them. Examples include medical or social models of disability, theories about how evidence should be collected, or theories about leadership and management. Equally, theories of practice development and 'what works' will shape the way projects are conducted and to what extent service users are enabled to participate. Although it may not always be easy to declare theoretical considerations in a way that includes service users, it may be possible to be explicit about the assumptions they give rise to.

Conclusion

Ethical issues in service user involvement are intricately linked to power, voice and empowerment. Different interpretations of what user involvement means in practice can lead to tensions concerning its goal and purpose and can leave service users disempowered. It is usually professionals and service managers who decide how service users are involved in development and this may limit the changes and improvement that can be achieved. Empowerment is not about the abandonment of leadership, but a process through which people can take control over their own lives, which is a goal aspired to in many recent policy documents. Yet there continues to be a lack of clarity about how user involvement is linked to policy objectives and what is hoped to be achieved by it in practical terms. Finally, practice developers who engage users in their work have a responsibility to produce more evidence and critically analyse the improvements user involvement is suggested to bring. Of course, the lack of evidence and analysis does not mean that there is not a positive effect. Yet if user participation is about the state's accountability to those for whom services in health and social care are provided then evidence about different forms of participation, their processes and outcomes must be scrutinized by both service users and providers.

Key points

- It is important that user involvement is not seen as an entity whose existence and definition can be taken for granted. There is a need for a better understanding about

how the policy of user involvement is interpreted in public service organizations and
how these interpretations shape how user involvement is put into practice.

- User involvement can be conceived as either a 'means to an end' or as an 'end in
itself.' The former is essentially target-oriented with the aim of containing costs and
promoting efficiency and best practice, whereas in the latter user involvement is
valued irrespective of tangible outcomes.
- While there is wide agreement among professionals in health and social care about
the importance of the involvement of users of services in decisions about their own
care or treatment options, their participation at a strategic level of service
improvements and developments is more controversial.
- User involvement can be seen from an economic perspective as consumer choice or
from a socio-political perspective as emancipatory and democratic. The way user
involvement is framed will have profound ethical implications for practitioners.
- Power is an important concept in relation to user involvement. Professionals and
service users are traditionally positioned in particular relationships with each other
as a result of how they are defined by, for example, in terms of social status and
knowledge, producing certain discourses which prescribe rules for judging what is
acceptable or inappropriate, what statements are true and which are false. Power is
exercised through these discourses.
- The following principles are useful when considering ethical conduct in user
involvement: clarity and transparency, empowerment, identity, commitment to
change, respect, equality and diversity, accountability and theoretical assumptions.

Useful links

Involve (national organization to support and promote active public involvement in
NHS, public health and social care research). Available online at www.invo.org.uk/.

References

Beresford, P. (2002) User involvement in research and evaluation: liberation or
    regulation? *Social Policy and Society*, 1(2): 95–105.
Crawford, M.J., Rutter, D., Manley, C., et al. (2002) *British Medical Journal*, 325: 1263–8.
Daykin, N., Rimmer, J., Turton, P. et al. (2002) Enhancing user involvement through
    interprofessional education in healthcare: the case of cancer services, *Learning in
    Health and Social Care*, 1(3): 122–31.
Department of Health (DoH) (2007) *A Dialogue of Equals: The Pacesetter Programme
    Community Engagement Guide*. London: DoH.
Department of Health (DoH) (2008a) *Stronger Voice, Better Care*. London: DoH.
Department of Health (DoH) (2008b) *Trans: A Practical Guide for the NHS*. London: DoH.
Department of Health (DoH) and British Institute of Human Rights (2008) *Human
    Rights in Healthcare: A Framework for Local Action*. London: DoH.
Evans, S., Tritter, J., Barley, V. et al. (2003) User involvement in UK cancer services:
    bridging the policy gap, *European Journal of Cancer Care*, 12: 331–8.
Faulkner, A. (2004) *The Ethics of Survivor Research: Guidelines for the Ethical Conduct of*

Research Carried Out By Mental Health Service Users and Survivors. Bristol: The Policy Press.

Foucault, M. (1980) Two lectures, in C. Gordon (ed.) *Power/Knowledge*. Brighton: Harvester Press, pp. 80–105.

Fudge, N., Wolfe, C.D.A. and McKevitt, C. (2008) Assessing the promise of user involvement in health service development: ethnographic study, *British Medical Journal*, 336: 313–17.

Haigh, C. (2008) Exploring the evidence base of patient involvement in the management of health care services, *Journal of Nursing Management*, 16: 452–62.

Harrison, S., Dowswell, G. and Milewa, T. (2002) Guest editorial: public and user involvement in the UK National Health Service, *Health and Social Care in the Community*, 10(2): 63–6.

Kotecha, N., Fowler, C. Donskoy, A.L., Johnson, P., Shaw, T. and Doherty, K. (2007) *A Guide to User-focused Monitoring: Setting Up and Running a Project*. London: The Sainsbury Centre for Mental Health.

Mills, S. (1997) *Discourse*. London: Routledge.

Mosquera, M., Zapata, Y., Lee, K., Arango, C. and Varela, A. (2001) Strengthening user participation through health sector reform in Columbia: a study of institutional change and social representation, *Health Policy and Planning*, 16 (Suppl. 2): 52–60.

Patterson, S., Weaver, T., Agath, K. et al. (2008) 'They can't solve the problems without us': a qualitative study of stakeholder perspectives on user involvement in drug treatment services in England, *Health and Social Care in the Community*, 17(1): 54–62.

Turner, B.S. (1997) From governmentality to risk, some reflections on Foucault's contribution to medical sociology, in A.R. Peterson and R. Bunton (eds) *Foucault, Health and Medicine*. Abingdon: Routledge.

Whittle, S., Turner, L. and Al-Alami, M. (2007) *Engendered Penalties: Transgender and Transsexual People's Experiences of Inequality and Discrimination, The Equalities Review*, February: 77. Available online at www.pfc.org.uk/files/EngenderedPenalties.pdf (accessed 12 February 2009).

9

Developing excellent service user engagement: a practical example

Melanie McSherry and Claire Brewis

Introduction

This chapter outlines the drivers for including users of services in the development of practice, both in a clinical and educational setting. Exploration is given to some of the ways in which this may be achieved and the ways in which some of the practical barriers to inclusion can be overcome. This chapter refers to 'service users' by using a generic term; it includes any person who accesses any type of health and social care service. Frequently, service users and carers are linked together and may be seen to have similar needs; however, for the purpose of this chapter, the specific issues around engaging carer involvement will not be considered as this is covered in Chapter 7. This chapter builds on the ideas and concepts offered in Chapters 7 and 8 by remaining focused on highlighting practical examples where service user engagement has taken place.

Background

Why engage users of service in health and social care practice development and education? Historically, the Community Health Councils (CHCs) (1974–2003) were established to fulfil a monitoring role of the National Health Service (NHS), which included advising the public and monitoring their complaints (DoH, 2008). The implementation the NHS Plan (DoH, 2000) replaced the CHCs with the Patient Advice and Liaison Services (PALS), who acted, among other things, as a key interface to provide feedback from service users to service staff. A culture of being receptive to patient feedback was encouraged, presenting a number of opportunities for service users, their relatives and carers, to influence services (DoH, 2007). It seems a logical extension of this philosophy of engagement for those institutions responsible for the education of tomorrow's health and social care workforce to embrace a similar influence and include users and carers to shape developments. Indeed, the directive to hear the 'user voice' is gaining momentum and is evident in numerous Department of Health (DoH) publications dating from the late 1990s, such as *Making a Difference: Strengthening the Nursing, Midwifery and Health Visiting Contribution to Health and Healthcare* (DoH, 1999), *The NHS Plan: A Plan for Investment. A Plan for Reform* (DoH, 2000), *Involving Patients and the Public in Healthcare* (DoH, 2001) and *Patient and Public Involvement (PPI): The Future Picture* (DoH, 2003). In light of these publications there have been initiatives undertaken within health and social care practice to facilitate hearing the service user voice. Current initiatives based within trust organizations are the Patient and Public Involvement Forums (PPIFs) that have now been replaced by the Local Involvement Networks (LINks). These developments are vitally important for service development and should be reflected in health and social care educational programmes and curriculum design, delivery and management.

In conjunction with this, the professionals moving out of the educational establishments and into service delivery should be in tune with the policy agenda and deliver meaningful health and social care. Indeed, health and social care education in England is bound, as part of quality assurance processes, to listen to what people think students in health and social care education should know and be involved in checking that this is actually happening (Quality Assurance Agency, 2006). Similarly, the Skills for Care organization, responsible for the modernization of social care education, is explicit in its engagement of users and carers (Skills for Care, 2008). It is widely accepted that health and social care educational programmes must produce qualified practitioners with the knowledge and skills to provide highly efficient care; in other words, we need to develop practitioners who are fit for practice. For students to develop these essential skills, the programme should link educational theory with relevant practical skills based up real-life situations and contexts. Therefore, educators must be in tune with clinical developments and trends to appreciate the context that students and qualified practitioners work in.

It is also imperative that the educator is aware of the political landscape influencing health and social care. An example of this would be the growing need for service providers to demonstrate that service users are involved in shaping service delivery. This is perhaps most evident in mental health service provision. Nick Clegg, leader for the Liberal Democrat party, has focused on mental health service provision and in particular has identified that 'A truly people centred NHS must empower patients so they have a real say in their own treatment' (Clegg, 2008: 16). He goes on to suggest that 'There is no reason why mental health service users should not have more choice over the options available to them and greater say in their care' (p. 17). This would be in partnership with the health and social care professionals involved with user. This opinion is also reflected across other health and social care settings; for example, stroke services, older people services and community-based services for the management of long-term conditions.

It is emphasized that best practice establishes a culture of engagement and

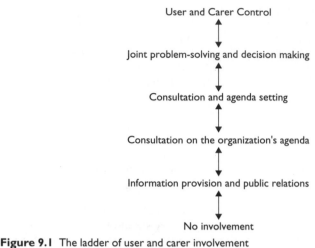

Figure 9.1 The ladder of user and carer involvement

Source: Adapted from Goss and Miller (1995)

partnership with users as opposed to a tokenistic gesture. Goss and Miller suggest adopting a ladder of user and carer involvement, (see Figure 9.1) the bottom rung representing 'no involvement', moving through more sharing of power through consultation, to a top rung of user and carer control (Goss and Miller, 1995.

The model was further adapted for mental health carer involvement in educational programmes (NCMH, 2003) (Table 9.1) and can equally apply to user and carer involvement in other professional disciplines and fields of practice. In this adapted model 'no involvement' would suggest a curriculum that is planned and delivered with no consultation of service users and carers being of the lowest value, against one of collaboration and partnership where there is joint decision-making and users and carers working as lecturers with appropriate reimbursement being of the highest value.

The attainment of the 'Partnership' level or the level of user and carer control is not without challenges to the practice and educational establishment and support mechanisms can take time and careful planning to be implemented. Consideration is given here to a number of ways in which engagement can be enhanced and further achieved.

Support mechanisms

Initiatives that require a change of culture in an organization are more likely to succeed with departmental management support. Ways of moving forward the organization and its culture with regard to practice development issues are well documented by McSherry and Warr (2008). Value and vision clarification for members of the organization or team are also important and can help

Table 9.1 Goss and Miller's ladder of user and carer involvement applied to mental health education

Level	Involvement	Characteristics
1	No involvement	The curriculum is planned, delivered and managed with no consultation or involvement of users
2	Passive involvement	User involvement is based on the discretion of the educationalist. Consultation of user views is through a third party. Limited occasional input in planning, delivery and/or management of the programme
3	Token involvement	Consultation with users is through non-decision-making forums. The content of the programme is defined by the organization rather than in response to user views. Users are involved in regular sessional input to the planning, delivery and/or management of the programme
4	Collaboration	Collaboration with users by listening to their views and accounts of issues and problems: these form the basis for decisions. Users are routinely involved in two of the following areas: planning, delivery and/or management of the programme
5	Partnership	Educationalists and users work together systematically, strategically, with full support, reimbursement structures and with education and training opportunities available. Users are involved at all stages of the planning, delivery and management processes. Decisions are made jointly. Users are involved in the assessment of students in the practice area. Users are working as lecturers

Source: Goss and Miller (1995)

focus any future strategic direction as detailed in Chapter 1. The culture change is more likely to succeed with team members being clear about how they fit into any future way of working, rather than a 'top-down' approach being imposed on them. McSherry and Warr (2008: 63) in an exercise on clarifying vision and values suggest it can assist individuals in thinking about the engagement of users and how and why to engage them in practice.

Activity 9.1 Reflective question

Before beginning to develop a strategic plan for innovation and change where user engagement is required, consider the following questions, both as an individual and by comparison with other team members. You may find these will aid the process:

- What are the aim(s) of the service?
- How do I contribute?
- What would an ideal service look like?
- What are my (our) values?

- What are my (our) vision(s)?
- How does our service relate to targets?
- How do we compare to best practice standards?

Read on and compare your answers with the rest of the chapter.

Developing a strategy for user engagement

Once discussion has taken place around what the organization hopes to achieve and where it would go to in relation to engaging users, developing a strategy with an action plan and SMART objectives (Table 9.2) is imperative. The primary author remains unknown but is believed to be derived from the seminal works of Drucker (1954). Using SMART objectives can be an effective way to take things forward. Any evolving strategy should be centred on promoting a culture that positively engages users and carers in the organization, be it an area of clinical practice or health and social care education.

Table 9.2 Smart objective setting

Acronym	Abbreviation	Rationale
S	Specific	Objectives should be precise in what it aims to achieve
M	Measurable	Objectives must be achievement focused so they can be quantified, rather than claiming to merely 'improve' on a particular aspect
A	Agreed	Objectives should be phrased in terms to allow all concerned to working to the same end
R	Realistic	Objectives that are phrased in simple and realistic way are likely to be achieved
T	Time-limited	Objectives must be time-limited in terms of declaring when you hope to achieve it by

The strategy should aim to reach the higher levels of engagement to that of 'partnership' working with users and carers, where the culture is one of automatic involvement of users and carers at all stages of the planning, delivery, management and evaluation of practice and learning, rather than tokenistic. Depending on where an organization is already in terms of engagement, it will determine the action points to be drawn up and the timescale in which they are to be addressed. Any such strategy must secure the support of management and team members in order to succeed as the task of developing such a culture across programmes successfully is huge if not already in place. It may be appropriate to ring-fence staff time in order to put in place the support infrastructure for such a venture, if there is currently no process for such as payment for involvement, induction or the storage of user and carer details.

Of course, the strategy should ideally engage users throughout all stages of development from the initial idea, proposal, and development, implementation and evaluation along with the sharing and dissemination and it would be best to take time to consider how you are going to do this by developing the best strategy.

C **Activity 9.2 Reflective question: how do we engage users at this stage?**

Consider the following at the stage of pulling together your user engagement strategy:

- Who are our users?
- What contacts does the organization already have in terms of user engagement?
- Can I draw on any of these contacts to help construct/validate our strategy?
- Do our users currently have any representative or support groups in the local area that we can approach for engagement?
- What contacts do people already have in the organization who may be appropriate to engage?

Read on and compare your answers with the rest of the chapter.

Strategic planning and management: the importance of establishing a working or steering group

Establishing a committee or steering/working group to consider any such project gives a focused approach and allows the sharing of ideas from different perspectives. Any committee is of course best served with representation from users or carers themselves, rather than assumptions being made and engagement at the lower levels of the NCMH adapted scale.

But where do we find people who are representative and not people who have things to get off their chest?

This is a question that is often asked by team members when such an issue is being driven forward. The answer may be that we can never find anyone who is wholly representative of users and carers and that those 'things that people want to get off their chest' may well have a message for consideration. What is more important is that committee members or contributors are varied in their representation and any action plans consider this variety at a strategic level. Establishing terms of reference for any committee can assist in drawing people back to the business and issues to be addressed.

Case study 9.1 An example from an educational setting: University of Teesside's School of Health and Social Care devised a set of terms of reference for user engagement

The School of Health and Social Care devised terms of reference for their user/carer engagement sub-committee once a strategy had been established. The sub-committee had membership from academic staff as well as users and carers and met once every academic term. The terms reflected how the sub-committee fed into the governance of the organization.

TERMS OF REFERENCE

1 To support the implementation of a coherent School of Health and Social Care user/carer engagement strategy.
2 To identify the resources and support mechanisms needed to support the strategy.
3 To promote the dissemination of good practice in the development and implementation of user/carer engagement action plans.
4 To support the self-assessment of user/carer engagements across the School's subject groups and consider issues arising from this.
5 Liaise with programme teams to generate and implement appropriate subject group and cross-subject group user/carer engagement plans.
6 To consider, address and feedback on user/carer engagement issues raised by the School committees, the student body and external reviewers.

There may be some further practical considerations in the running of a committee or group that involves users and carers. You may need to consider if there are access barriers associated with the meeting room, such as stairs or circulation space in the room. Notes may need to be translated to Braille but this can easily be overcome by finding a local service for this and establishing a relationship with them. Suitable parking close to venue may also be a consideration.

Establishing a baseline of current engagement

Auditing the current engagement of users in practice and programmes is important to establish a strategic direction and can facilitate the sharing of good practice among colleagues. A popular method is by self-audit and some tools already exist to assist with this in the education field; for example, the Trent NHS Strategic Health Authority (2005) and NCMH (2003). Whatever your field of practice, you can construct your own by breaking down the different aspects of the service provision into your domains of practice.

Based on Activity 9.3 Table 9.3 offers some possible areas for your audit.

↻ **Activity 9.3 Reflective questions: areas of our practice that a user could become involved in**

Consider the following questions in constructing your self-audit form:

- What are different elements of service provision?
- What are the development needs of staff?
- What are the different elements of service for the people we serve?
- How do we consult others on how we do things currently?
- In what areas can we expand this?

You may want to compare your answers with the section below.

Table 9.3 Possible areas for user engagement audit

Practice	Education of health and social professionals
• Recruitment and training of staff • Service development and planning of services • Evaluating current services • Dealing with complaints	• Selection of students • Curriculum design • Approval of new programmes • Delivering the curriculum • Assessment of student performance • Evaluating effectiveness of programmes

Once you have established the domains of your practice, you can audit your service to establish where you currently engage users and identify the areas for development. These areas of development can be worked into an action plan for further engagement. Having prioritized the key areas for consideration prior to implementation of a user engagement, a major consideration is staff development and support.

Staff development and support

First, awareness raising of the policies and any strategies in practice around engaging users and carers is an essential factor to the success of this agenda. Second, knowledge of the support available in how to progress the strategy in everyday work is essential. Methods of communicating this to staff will need to be established, either through regular communications, announcements and newsletters or more formalized training opportunities. Further information associated with communication is outlined in Chapter 1.

Some staff may have concerns about finding users who are appropriate and representative as well as how to support them in the activities. Procedures already in place, such as payment policies and induction, need to be advertised. A good infrastructure in the organization to support staff can assist considerably. For example, if a payment policy and procedure is established, alongside a database of appropriate users who have undergone an induction process, it will perhaps go some way in supporting a keen yet unsure member of staff in inviting a user into the classroom to share their experiences where education or training is taking place. Figure 9.2 outlines the infrastructure requirements for supporting staff in engaging users.

• A database of people recruited/willing to engage

• Establishing a payment policy to reward users for their time

• Contacts with organizations that can translate written materials to Braille

• A staff member with dedicated time to recruit users and brief them around issues of engagement

• Including any strategy awareness raising in the induction of new staff

Figure 9.2 An infrastructure that will support staff in engaging users

A range of opportunities exist for staff development and support to facilitate understanding and application of the principles of user and carer engagement. If the organization has an individual with dedicated time to progress this agenda, their sharing and dissemination of information and meeting of individuals at team meetings can be a starting point. The agenda can be raised with new staff through induction processes. The sharing of good practice via learning and teaching seminars, professional forums and professional network to name but a few can encourage staff to adopt similar techniques and approaches. Workshops and conferences are available regionally and nationally, often tying in with the remit of local health and social care provision. Local primary care trusts will often have member reference groups to support their own role in engaging users of service while acute trusts will use local involvement networks or LINks (DoH, 2008)

Networking with local user and carer groups can be a valuable source of support for staff looking to expand their contacts. Often this may be a group linked to a staff member's clinical or practice background and attending a meeting can stimulate thinking and help break down barriers with regard to finding appropriate people to engage.

Induction and support for the users and carers

The users who agree to become involved will require some form of preparation for the activities you wish them to become involved in. Induction and training can take a number of guises, depending on the types of activity you would like to engage them with. Induction can vary from simple briefing around the organization and what it is hoping to achieve with their engagement to more formalized credit-bearing programmes of study that may appeal to some individual users and carers.

Case study 9.2 An example of a user and carer event in a university

Users and carers were invited to 'tell their story' to groups of students engaged in inter-professional learning within a university. An induction afternoon was held to introduce users and carers to:

- the aims of the event
- typically what they may expect
- what related activities the students would be engaged in
- confidentiality issues
- practical considerations such as timing, venue, refreshments
- meeting their facilitator and to give those involved an opportunity to voice any concerns or have queries answered.

Similar to Case study 9.2, another approach sometimes adopted in NHS trusts is to run induction around advocacy and ways in which users can feel able to use their experience of the service as a tool for improving service delivery.

User engagement: innovations in curriculum design, delivery, management and evaluation of the education of health and social care professionals

This section specifically explores the notion of involving service users in curriculum design, delivery, management and evaluation as well as the assessment of student learning. The overarching philosophical guidelines are reviewed in the light of recommended good practice and then examples are given of how an organization might attempt to involve service users in educational and assessment processes. The aim is to highlight the practical aspects so that the reader might consider the relevance for their own particular situation and be encouraged to facilitate service users' contribution.

Importance of involving service users in educational programmes

It is widely accepted that health and social care educational programmes must produce qualified practitioners with the knowledge and skills to provide highly efficient care. In other words, we need to develop health and social care professionals who are fit for practice. For students to develop these essential skills, the programme should link educational theory with relevant practical skills based on real-life situations and contexts. Therefore, educators must be in tune with clinical developments and trends to appreciate the context that students and qualified practitioners work in.

Selecting students appropriately for professional educational programmes

We must remember that the professional interviewing of students for their programme sees the applicant through the eyes of who will make a good student as well as an assumption as to who will work best in practice alongside practice colleagues. However, the user can provide a different and valuable viewpoint identifying the attributes they would like a health or social care professional to hold if they were involved in their care. Lecturers often assume that engaging users in the selection of their students will involve sitting on interview panels, which are often lengthy processes and often difficult to organize. This need not be the case, even if the interviewing of applicants is the agreed procedure for access to the programme of study. For those who do wish to engage users on interview panels induction and support for the user will be required beforehand and this is achievable with careful planning. However, alternative methods can be employed as follows:

Engagement in drawing up selection criteria

Can be done by consultation of individual users and carers or visiting established local support groups, allowing them to suggest, shape and refine the admissions criteria.

Question setting

Users and carers can be consulted on appropriate questions to be asked of applicants and desired responses sought. If the admissions procedure involves group discussion some topical and pertinent scenarios for group discussion can be put forward by individuals or groups of users and carers. For example, on an occupational therapy programme, Stockton Parent Support for families and special needs groups put forward a variety of topics for use at group interview such as:

The emphasis in education for people with learning disabilities is on life skills rather than reading and writing, etc. Is this the appropriate approach?

Often therapists meeting parents of disabled children for the first time receive an angry reaction. Why may this be so? Discuss.

Reviewing the procedure for admissions

Using the expertise of users and carers as active members of programme boards or advisory groups.

In addition to the above, the utilization of information technology (IT) and patient narratives are becoming a popular resource. These are readily available via the Internet and can be employed as part of a task or focal point for discussion at interview. Alternative media can be employed such as video or DVD. For example, a social work team commissioned a group of actors with disabilities to produce a series of scenarios on DVD that can be utilized in either teaching or the interview process.

How to involve service users in curriculum design: practical application

In order to engage with service users when designing a curriculum, it is important at the outset that the curriculum development team have clarity of what is expected of each person/representative. However, the process should also start with a 'blank sheet of paper' rather than with a preconceived idea of what the end product will look like. If a philosophy of the programme is to develop students' knowledge and skills to engage with service users as equal partners in decision-making, embracing the aim to achieve a patient-led NHS, then the same principles should be applied to the curriculum development strategy. The contribution of each representative must be recognized and valued from the beginning. There are several practical aspects to consider when seeking service users' views/consultation or participation as a group member especially if sustainability of the group is required.

First, identify the stakeholders who can make a positive contribution specific to the educational programme. In other words, the service user should have some understanding of the service context that the students will experience. For example, a service user who has experience of physiotherapy services at home may not be the best representative for a pre-registration children's nursing programme. Furthermore, one service user may not be representative for a number of programmes. It may be necessary to draw service users from a wide variety of backgrounds. The need to consider where to draw service user representatives from could prove to be a difficult issue. Including service users from established organizations rather than relying on isolated individuals may also help with support for the individual and could also increase consistency with representation. The most likely way to identify potential service user representatives could be by way of informal networks. Often clinical educationalists have links with ex-patient groups or established support group networks. Alternatively, links with senior health or social care staff could be the initial starting point for gaining access to self-help groups or other support groups. Access to service user groups may take more time than initially estimated and getting suitable representation is vitally important.

Second, a major consideration will be payment issues that must be robust and recognize the service user as an expert consultant, demonstrating value of the contribution. It may be that service users will decline payments offered if they impact on benefit claims but this should not deter offering payment. The service user may ask for payment to be made to charity funds or other alternatives instead. Some service users may need or prefer to be paid cash on the day of attendance.

Thought will need to be given for other practical aspects of involving service users in educational curriculum development, such as the need for service users' attendance at meetings. Where service users are required to attend meetings, the environment and resources must be accessible; this includes the building structure as well as materials such as documentation and information. Again, it should be clear at the outset how frequent meetings will be, duration and if comfort breaks will be given. Some service users may also need assistance from their care staff and their needs should be taken into account.

With regard to the philosophy of embracing true service user involvement, it is important to ensure that different service user groups are not discriminated against; for example, black and ethnic minority groups, deaf or blind service users. When considering resources, thought might be needed in providing additional support such as texts in Braille and translators for non-English-speaking service users. The transport needs to and from the meeting place should be taken into account and potential difficulties should be resolved to ensure that service users are able to contribute effectively without being concerned about logistical matters. The way that meetings are arranged could influence service user involvement; for example, if meetings are scheduled too early service users may be put off attending. It may be possible to consult with service user groups and then inform the rest of the curriculum planning team of the feedback. This might resolve attendance difficulties but this could be at the expense of service users being fully engaged in dialogue during meetings. There is also a potential that the information is unintentionally 'filtered' through the messenger.

Where service users are invited to attend meetings, ground rules for being involved might be useful. For example, if service users commit to the curriculum development project, would they then be obliged to attend every meeting for the duration of the project? The way in which the meeting is conducted should be comfortable for all participants and if the manner is formal, service users need to be made aware of the etiquette such as turning mobile phones to silent. It would be akin to new members of staff being inducted into the organizational norms and educational and clinical jargon should be avoided.

The inclusion of service users in programme management

Goss and Miller (1995) encourage joint decision-making with users of service in their proposed ladder of involvement. Part of this decision-making can be in the form of ensuring that service users are involved in approving educational programmes and able to sanction a curriculum that meets their requirements. This can be a departure from tradition within universities but by no means impossible to achieve. The existing approval process may need to be adapted to allow this to happen and briefing will need to be given to both users invited to be approved panel members and the chair of any panel, so as they acknowledge the role of the user on the panel and consideration is given to their needs. Good practice is to draw up briefing materials for those concerned about what to expect and what form the process will take. An example of what to include in a briefing sheet for users invited to be an approval panel members:

- **What is the event?**
- **What is the process?**
- **What is the time commitment?**
- **Who will be there?**
- **How can you contribute?**
- **What can you do if you don't understand something?**
- **What are the domestic arrangements?**

Programme management involves a range of activities that can present opportunities for engaging users, besides approval of the actual university programme.

Involving service users in delivery of programme content

There are numerous ways of involving service users in delivering course content. The type of programme will influence the method of involving service users. For example, a pre-registration nursing programme might have 250 students in one cohort where a postgraduate occupational therapy programme might have 20 students per cohort. It is essential at the outset to identify the learning aims and outcomes for students and to match the content delivery to these aims. Resources such as lecture room availability for large numbers will affect provision.

Activity 9.4 Reflective questions

Identify the advantages and disadvantages for each method for the student, service user and teacher

- Single service user presentation such as key lecture.
- Service user facilitation of small group discussion.
- Drama presentation by a group of service users.
- DVD or website presentation and discussion.
- Audiotape presentation and discussion.
- Written accounts/patient narratives.

Read on and compare your answers with the remainder of the chapter.

Reflecting on Activity 9.3, it would appear that overall responsibility for managing the training/teaching session should remain with the course teacher and the individual needs of the service user should be taken into account. Preparation should be considered, as it is essential to identify practical aspects such as whether or not the service user will respond to questions from the group (which may be more invasive than expected). It may be necessary to include a debrief session with the service user following a session if they feel vulnerable, emotional or exposed following the experience. Students might also be affected by the experience and need additional support from appropriate staff. The nature of health and social care might mean that very personal issues are explored and guidance about confidentiality should be given. For example, service users might be offended to know that students have discussed their presentation with people who are not participants on the programme and this should be reviewed prior to the interaction.

For large cohort numbers, consistency of presentation might be an issue and the use of DVD or website/audiotape or written account material can be helpful. There are service user groups who will often agree to participate in producing material if commissioned by the educational institution. This could include health or social care scenarios acted out or drama group presentations showing positive interventions and/or poor outcomes. The benefit of using these resources will be that all students have access to the same teaching at the same time, thus reducing inequity.

User engagement in the assessment of learning

According to the Trent Strategic Health Authority (2005), it is essential to have 'systematic, explicit and formalised processes to support service user and carer involvement in assessment' (p. 28). However, the processes must also reflect the local context and evolve from the educational infrastructure. Every area will have specific needs and may seek to involve service users in a wide variety of ways. It is important to recognize that what may be appropriate for one locality may not be suitable for another and because one method works well for one institution, it is unlikely that the same method can be successfully transposed to a different situation. In other words, there is no 'one size fits all' solution to involving service users in the assessment of learning. Indeed, within one organization different processes may be needed depending up the learning experience under assessment.

The way in which assessment takes place in clinical settings will vary depending up the programme and service setting. Many educational institutions will support clinical staff, practice mentors, to assess students during the placement. Frequently, students are required to self-assess during placement experiences. In other areas, academic staff might also be involved in both formally and informally assessing the student alongside the practice mentor in a tripartite meeting (Figure 9.3) The notion of service users being involved in student assessment is a relatively new concept.

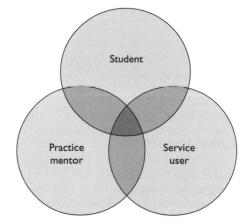

Figure 9.3 The tripartite arrangement

There have been few recent examples in the literature of service user involvement with assessing learning although there would appear to be acceptance that service users ought to be involved in direct assessment of student learning. Speers (2008: 113) makes the point that an increase in consumerism and a recognition that some health service users have a deeper understanding of their own needs than professionals has led to educational institutions considering the way forward. In her study undertaken in 2005, Speers investigated the opinions of stakeholders including mental health service users, student nurses, ex-student nurses, practice mentors and lecturers using interview methodology. The potential advantages for student nurses and future care provision was highlighted against the potential disadvantages for the students. A summary of the advantages and disadvantages of service user involvement in assessment are outlined in Table 9.4.

User engagement in programme development, curriculum design, management and assessment of learning is a new innovative and creative approach to educational provision. The challenge for health and social care professionals is in maximizing its potential in the future.

User engagement: the way forward for the future

Gould (2008: p25) refers to patient choice for service users for mental health care. In this article he quotes Liz Felton, chief executive of the charity Together, who advocates that 'people who use mental health services to take a leadership role in designing them'. She goes on to suggest that 'If health services are to promote service user leadership, it is important that those services can demonstrate that they contribute to improving "quality of life" outcome measures'. The notion of service users taking a leadership role is significant and warrants further consideration.

Table 9.4 Advantages and disadvantages of service user involvement in assessment

Advantages	Disadvantages
Service users' views	*Service users' views*
• Enhanced student learning	• Students could be demoralized
• Better care	• Feedback might not be fair/honest
• Empowerment/respect for service users	• Lack of confidentiality/anonymity
• Stronger validity of assessment as service users have the best sense of the quality of a therapeutic relationship	might cause problems
Nurses' views	*Nurses' views*
• Potential of unmediated feedback enhancing student confidence	• Students could be demoralized or judged unfairly
• Benefit to assessment validity of better triangulated evidence	• Possible unreliability of mental health service user assessment due to mental state
• Enhanced student learning	• Service users are not trained to give constructive feedback
• Philosophical 'fit' with service user empowerment/collaborative working	• Potential harm done to service users through coercion, fear and/or burden of responsibility
• Could result in a therapeutic 'knock-on effect' for service users	

Source: Adapted from Speers (2008)

Case study 9.3 Interpersonal development

Student nurse, Amy Jones, has been on the ward for six weeks. She is now familiar with the ward routine and has a good understanding of the client group's needs. She usually works two spans of duty with her mentor, staff nurse Carter and one shift with her associate mentor. While Amy enjoys working with staff nurse Carter and is encouraged to develop her knowledge and skills, she struggles with her interpersonal communication with patients when not directly supervised. For example, she becomes easily flustered when dealing with individual needs of the patient and may appear abrupt or grumpy. When working with her associate mentor, Amy is left to work alongside support staff with minimal direct supervision. This illustrates the different perspectives that might be held about Amy's clinical performance.

• Do you think that the mentors might view Amy differently?
• How might Amy rate her own performance?
• What opinions do you think the patients or families might hold?

The assessment of the student should be an equal partnership between student self-assessment, practice mentor assessment based on direct observation and service user assessment based on personal experience with the student.

Traditionally, the medical practitioner or consultant was seen as the lead in deciding the medical care for the patient. Often decisions were made in conjunction with other members of the health care team such as the nurses, physiotherapists, occupational therapists, social workers and others frequently without the patient being present. There was an obvious hierarchy in clinical decision-making (see Figure 9.4).

The notion of the patient or service user taking a lead in deciding what is best for them challenges the traditional concept of health care. This may be seen to reflect the changes in society whereby service users are more informed about health care options and more willing to act as a consumer of health care services. It is important to think about the range of clinical decisions that affect the service user, so while treatment and medication prescriptions might be seen to rate as highly important, other decisions could equally be seen as impacting in a significant way for the individual service user. The involvement of the service user in decision-making in any treatment plan is personal to that individual. Within local practice settings, service users are often invited to senior nurse meetings to discuss their experiences of service provision to help inform staff of their experiences. This can be a very effective strategy to help identify examples of positive experiences as well as recognizing potential areas for developing the service provision. It is important to understand what constitutes excellent service user involvement in order to strive to achieve it for every person as outlined in Case study 9.4.

In considering this case study, the acronym ASSIST might be useful as a model to base user engagement around:

A   Audit current activity of service engagement
S   Strategy development with organizational commitment
S   Support for staff and resource development
I   Infrastructure support
S   Seize the opportunity and be proactive
T   Take time to develop relationships

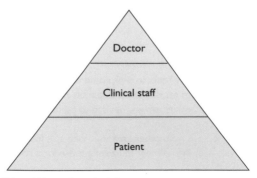

Figure 9.4 Traditional hierarchy principle

Case study 9.4 An example of an effective episode in a case study of service user engagement

Mrs Jones has been in hospital for three weeks following a fall at home. She is due to go home in two days time and is slightly anxious about how she will cope. Mrs Jones agrees with medical staff that she is now medically fit and her medication has been reviewed with her, resulting in her taking fewer tablets. With Mrs Jones's agreement, the nurse and occupational therapist discuss the recent home visit made with Mrs Jones to her house in preparation for her safe discharge. Some recommendations are highlighted to reduce recurrence of another fall. For example, Mrs Jones had some difficulty in carrying a cup of tea to her living room while using her walking stick. The occupational therapist suggests that the rug be removed from the hallway as it could be a trip hazard. Mrs Jones and her daughter are asked to consider the acceptability of this.

Conclusion

Service user engagement may be seen from a macro perspective as a directive for clinical services and educationalists to take on board. Alternatively, if viewed positively, it can be an opportunity to enrich the relationship between people providing a service and those people receiving the service. Each organization should consider the local context and shape the involvement to meet their needs. Perhaps the most important facet of engaging service users is to ensure that there is a solid infrastructure in place. This requires effort and energy to put into place support strategies for staff; for example, access to resources such as databases with contact details of potential contributors may be time consuming to establish but will be invaluable to educators who want to invite service users into the classroom. The messages from service users are important and while the experience will be unique to them, the experience account can be applied to many different clinical contexts both within health care environments and at home.

Key points

- Involving service users in clinical and educational developments should be seen as an opportunity to get the 'expert opinion' on how to shape services.
- Energy and enthusiasm are needed to build a secure infrastructure that will support service user involvement.
- Learn lessons from other areas but 'one size fits all' are unlikely to be successful. The service user involvement must reflect the local context and be owned by the collective.
- Investing time in making resources available will reap rewards.

- Where face-to-face contact is not possible, there are a range of alternative ways for involving service users, such as DVD and audiotape material, website and narrative accounts.
- Monitoring of involvement is useful to demonstrate how well the organization is facilitating and embedding service user involvement in the cultural fabric.

References

Clegg, N. (2008) We shall bring mental health under our wing, *Health Service Journal*, 11 September, pp.16–17.

Department of Health (DoH) (1999) *Making a Difference: Strengthening the Nursing, Midwifery and Health Visiting Contribution to Health and Healthcare*. London: Her Majesty's Stationery Office.

Department of Health (DoH) (2000) The *NHS Plan: A Plan for Investment, a Plan for Reform*. London: DoH.

Department of Health (DoH) (2001) *Involving Patients and the Public in Healthcare: A Discussion Document*. London: Her Majesty's Stationery Office (HMSO).

Department of Health (DoH) (2003) *Patient and Public Involvement (PPI): The Future Picture*. London: DoH.

Department of Health (DoH) (2007) *PALS*. Available online at www.dh.gov.uk/en/ Managingyourorganisation/PatientAndPublicinvolvement/Patientadviceandliai sonservices/DH_4081305 (accessed 19 December 2009).

Department of Health (DoH) (2008) *Patient and Public Involvement*. Available online at www.dh.gov.uk/en/Managingyourorganisation/PatientAndPublicinvolvement/ DH_085874 (accessed 19 December 2008).

Drucker, P. (1954) *The Practice of Management*. London: Pan.

Goss, S., and Miller, C. (1995) *From Margin to Mainstream: Developing User and Carer-centred Community Care*. York: Joseph Rowntree Foundation.

Gould, M. (2008) Mental health: your shout, *Health Service Journal*, 11 September, pp. 25–31.

McSherry, R., and Warr, J. (2008) *An Introduction to Excellence in Practice Development in Health and Social Care*. Maidenhead: Open University Press.

Northern Centre for Mental Health (NCMH) (2003) *National Quality Continuous Improvement Tool for Mental Health Education*. Durham: NCMH.

Quality Assurance Agency (2006) *Quality Assurance Agency in Healthcare Education*. Available online at www.qaa.ac.uk/health/ (accessed 19 December 2008).

Skills for Care (2008) www.skillsforcare.org.uk/home/home.aspx.

Speers, J. (2008) Service user involvement in the assessment of practice competency in mental health, *Nursing Nurse Education in Practice*, 8: 112–19.

Trent NHS Strategic Health Authority (2005) *Principles for Practice Involving Service Users and Carers in Health Care Education and Training*. Mansfield: Trent SHA.

10

Equality and diversity in practice development

Sabi Redwood and Vanessa Heaslip

Introduction

The purpose of this chapter is to introduce you to important concepts and frameworks in relation to equality and diversity to enable you to reflect on your experiences of working with a diverse range of clients and colleagues. Within the broader context of policy, practice and service delivery in health and social care, you are asked to question and challenge your own attitudes that may help you become more aware of factors that can influence the way in which we work with clients and colleagues. Such a critical awareness is crucial with regard to practice development because change and innovation are directly and indirectly linked to assumptions, values and beliefs about other people.

Background

Practice development is about enabling health and social care workers to transform the culture and the context of care (McSherry and Warr, 2008; McCormack et al., 1999). It sets out actively to improve care and services by working with practitioners and the users of services to shape the way 'things are done' through processes of collaboration and engagement at individual, team and organizational level. While practice development is about promoting a culture that strives for excellence in care, it is important to remember that practice development is itself influenced by the broader culture and the context in which it takes place (Walsh and Moss, 2007).

How a society views all the different people who participate in it is an important aspect of its culture. The notion of human rights as well as values such as fairness, respect, autonomy, dignity and equality signal a commitment to a number of core rights that everyone is entitled to irrespective of their different cultural identities and needs. Legislation and policy, eliminating prejudice, oppression and unlawful discrimination has been an important vehicle for making human rights real in people's lives. For example, there are a number of statutory instruments that have a bearing on services in health and social care, both for the users of services and providers. They are the rights enshrined in the European Convention on Human Rights, adopted in the UK in 1998; the European Directives that prohibit discrimination on the grounds of religion or belief, disability, sexual orientation or ethnic origin with regard to accessing services and working conditions which, begun in 2003, have been phased in over several years; and the Equality Act 2006 that created the Equality and Human Rights Commission in the UK bringing together the six equality strands of gender, ethnic origin, disability, age, religion or faith and sexual orientation. The intention of this legislation has clearly been to introduce a culture of human rights into the public services. As Hunt (2004) points out, these laws signify a shift of emphasis away from simply outlawing discrimination to the positive duty to promote equality. However, she warns that these top-down initiatives are 'limited in their capacity to bring about a change in attitude and behaviour and cannot wipe out the cycle of socialization, entrenched values and practices that have formed the norms of our society for many years' (p. 412).

This set of human rights and equality legislation has had profound implications for health and social care. Since 2000, there have been a number of policy papers documenting key policy changes and developments for health and social care to ensure that service providers and workers comply with legal duties to tackle discrimination and promote equality. Similarly, current government policy has demonstrated a commitment towards the recognition of diversity in access to health and social care, the quality of care, the importance of a diverse workforce in health and social care and the links between these issues (DoH, 2000). These links are being explicitly articulated in terms of human rights that are used as principles on which to base health and social care policy, practice and service delivery. Not only is there a recognition that having one's human rights ignored leads to poor health, but also that their active promotion in public services, and health and social care in particular, is seen as instrumental to people's health and well-being (DoH and British Institute of Human Rights, 2008). Thus, there has been a shift of emphasis from protecting vulnerable and minority groups from discrimination to one of promoting the human rights of everyone. This notion is expressed in, for example, a guide on caring for transgender people: 'Individual care and respect begins with appreciating that all people are individuals. The National Health Service (NHS) is there for everyone, no matter in what way they are different' (DoH and British Institute of Human Rights, 2008: 20). This human rights-based approach to care is being introduced to improve service design and delivery for everyone and is based on the following principles:

- putting human rights principles and standards at the heart of policy and planning
- ensuring accountability
- empowerment
- participation and involvement
- non-discrimination and attention to vulnerable groups.

These principles must underpin any contribution to putting individual needs at the centre of decision-making processes. However, it is important to acknowledge that workers in health and social care should be enabled to move beyond compliance to legislation or memorizing their legal duty to avoid discrimination and promote equality. A checklist approach, which may be adopted in response to increased monitoring, demands for complaints and litigation processes and other bureaucratic procedures, will not be sufficient to ensure that human rights are being protected and promoted. Developing practice and striving for excellence in care demands that practitioners take moral responsibility for uncovering the harmful defences and denial that are likely to be part of their everyday reality, but are usually not recognized as contributing to systemic discrimination and oppression. This means having a heightened awareness of their own attitudes and assumptions and a willingness to appreciate differences, recognize common ground and challenge policies and practices that contravene people's human rights (Hunt, 2004).

This chapter explores these issues and looks in more detail at how discrimination operates in health and social care and how practitioners can use this knowledge to uncover and challenge inequality and discrimination.

Activity 10.1 Reflective question

Outline what you think is meant by the following terms:

- diversity
- equal opportunities
- equality
- equity
- human rights.

Compare your answers with the information in the following section.

Just political correctness?

The terms 'political correctness' and being 'politically correct' are usually identifications imposed on people by those who are politically opposed to attempts to change behaviour and the use of language that is sexist, racist or homophobic. Thus, people who seek to persuade organizations such as workplaces or public services to adopt guidelines that ask people to think about how they act and speak, to avoid certain behaviour and language, and to adopt alternatives have been ridiculed in certain media and discourses. On the other hand, simply changing the language we use clearly does not remove oppression or constitute social change. Interestingly, the changes in language to change identities, values and representations by introducing into public services terms such as 'flexibility' and 'individual responsibility' and extending market identities such as 'customer' or 'consumer' to health and social care and education have gone largely unnoticed as it has relied on the covert power of systems (Fairclough, 2003). As Hall (1999) points out, a political strategy that seeks to bring about social change needs to be integrated at a number of different levels. In relation to sexism, for example, this would have to include the eradication of sexist language as well as tackling salary inequalities or procedures for promotion that discriminate against female employees. Thus, the freedom from discrimination and oppression is an experience that must go beyond language. Yet we need to be clear about the language we use and how it might contribute to the experience of discrimination and oppression. In the following section we define the terms that are frequently used when we talk about social justice and fair treatment.

Diversity

Diversity focuses attention on the variety and differences inherent among individuals and groups from different multicultural backgrounds, experiences and approaches. Sometimes these differences are obvious as in race and skin colour and language, or physical disability. Sometimes they are implicit, as in beliefs and values. Sometimes they are simply hidden as in the case of sexuality. Within a culture of diversity, difference is valued positively and is seen to bring about benefits for society. The analogy that would describe a culture of diversity is that of the mosaic in which the differently coloured pieces make up a pattern or picture. Peoples' difference in identity and need require different approaches or treatment as service users or employees in order to achieve positive outcomes for themselves and for the organization (Douglas, 2004).

Equal opportunities

Equal opportunities is an approach predicated on the belief that if everyone is treated in the same way, fair practice and outcomes will be achieved. The emphasis is on the freedom from discrimination on the basis of sex, skin colour, age or disability. The approach embraces positive discrimination to redress past negative discrimination (Douglas, 2004). It is based on a legal framework and compliance is regularly monitored. The analogy that would describe the equal opportunities approach is that of a melting pot in which the ingredients in the pot are people of different identities, cultures, colours, religions, and so on. They combine to produce a new multi-ethnic society.

Equity

The term 'equity' is concerned with the notion of how resources, or indeed costs, are distributed. It refers to the fair distribution of opportunities and rewards and the fair imposition of costs and punishments. Thus, everyone should have equal access to education, for example, but people who earn more should pay higher taxes and people committing more serious offences should receive more severe prison sentences.

Equality

'Equality' refers to the idea that individuals' identity, skin colour, social and economic background and ethnic origin must have no bearing on the way they are treated in matters of justice and public life. This means that every individual is subject to the same laws and that no group or individual has any special privileges. It also implies that everyone has the same opportunities and chance to hold various positions in society on the basis of their efforts and achievements rather than on the basis of their socio-economic background.

Human rights

The term 'human rights' refers to a moral entitlement that is afforded to everyone on the basis of their humanity. Human rights apply to all people equally irrespective of identity, skin colour, social and economic background or nationality. They specify the minimum conditions for human dignity and a tolerable life. The preamble of the 1948 Declaration of Human Rights refers to a 'recognition of the inherent dignity and of the equal and inalienable rights of all members of the human family is the foundation of freedom, justice and peace in the world'. There is a distinction between absolute rights that may never be interfered with, not even in times of war or national emergency. Lack of resources is never an excuse for interfering with an absolute right. An example is Article 3 (the prohibition of torture, inhuman and degrading treatment). On the other hand, limited rights are not absolute. They may be limited in certain strictly defined circumstances. An example is Article 5 (the right to liberty and security). This right may be limited in circumstances where someone is lawfully detained on the basis that the person has committed a crime or is suffering from serious mental health problems (DoH and British Institute of Human Rights, 2008).

Discrimination and oppression in health and social care

The vision of an inclusive and human rights-based approach to policy making, workforce planning and staffing, service commissioning and delivery, and inclusive planning and public health strategy has set the tone for the development of practice. The 'Darzi Report' (DoH, 2008a) identified quality at the heart of the health service; this is reinforced by the development of core values of the NHS that include respect and dignity, commitment to quality of care, compassion, improving lives, workings together for patient and everyone counts. However, such vision stands little chance of becoming a real experience if we view the users of services and practitioner delivering these services as one-dimensional people who all have the same needs, or if we do not challenge our taken-for-granted ideas and assumptions about people who are different to us in terms of skin colour, age or cultural background. Professional bodies are working in concert with this vision: for example, The Code of Conduct for Nurses and Midwives (Nursing and Midwifery Council, 2008) and the Standards of Conduct, Performance and Ethics for Allied Health Professional (Health Professions Council, 2004) make it explicit that clients must be treated with respect and dignity and not discriminated against. However, there is evidence that discrimination and inequalities in health continue to be a major issue for many vulnerable groups. For example, Ashkam (2008: 41) reports in an evaluation of older people's use of services:

> On the principle of countering discrimination, [the projects] illustrated particularly well the tension between older age as a period of decline – about which it is thought not a lot can be done – and the more positive view of later life, with its active approach to meeting the needs of older service users. As long as some service providers continue to see older people in nihilistic or stereotyped ways, it may take more professional education or national policy directives (such as NHS-funded nursing care) to improve the situation for older people. . . . The situation is not helped by the perhaps inevitable tendency to 'typify' or place older people into cultural or medical categories rather than treating each person as an individual, with the consequent risk of stereotyping them and in so doing discriminating against them.

◠ Activity 10.2 Reflective question

Ashkam talks about older people being seen in stereotyped ways. Can you identify some of these negative stereotypes? Why are they harmful to people? What are your views about the period of old age?

Read the following section and compare your answers with the analysis of the case study.

In the following section, we introduce a framework to enable you to understand how discrimination and oppression can operate in health and social care. These processes are often unconscious; in other words, discriminatory practice is not necessarily intended or malicious. However, in order to develop practice in line with the principles of human rights-based care, it is important to bring these unhelpful assumptions and beliefs to a conscious level in order to articulate and understand them.

If you were to explore dictionary definitions of discrimination, you will see that it refers to the identification of difference, which could be either positive or negative. However, negative discrimination is often associated with the unfair or unequal treatment of individuals or groups by the alignment of

↻ **Activity 10.3 Reflective question**

Outline what you think is meant by the following terms:

- discrimination
- oppression
- covert
- overt.

Compare your answers with the information in the following section.

negative attributes (Thompson, 2001, 2003). Examples of this could be the perception that all young black men are violent and involved in gangs, or that all asylum-seekers are 'bogus' seeking to come to Britain for an easier life by living on benefits. When negative discrimination occurs, the resulting experience is generally one of oppression that Thompson (2001: 34) defines as 'inhuman or degrading treatment of individuals or groups; hardship and injustice brought about by the dominance of one group over another; and/or the negative and demeaning exercise of power'. While the word oppression often conjures up mental pictures of oppressive regimes in other countries, Young (1990) argues that it is being increasingly used to describe the disadvantage and injustice that some social groups experience, not necessarily because society actively seeks to disadvantage some groups of people (active oppression), but rather as a result of the unchallenged societal norms, laws and assumptions (passive oppression).

Discrimination and oppression can be seen to be linked to inequality in a number of different ways (Figure 10.1). To illustrate this, we use the example of votes for women in Edwardian Britain. During this time women did not

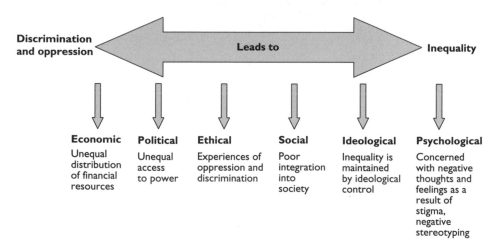

Figure 10.1 Mechanisms leading to inequality

have the same access to financial resources as men, either because they were poor or because it was socially expected that middle and upper-class married women did not work, but instead remained within the family home to rear children. This not only reduced the financial independence of women, but also their status within society. This inequality with men was reinforced at the political level as women did not receive the same rights to vote as men until 1928, and it was a further 30 years before women were allowed access to the House of Lords. This lack of representation of women's views led to legislation and policies that were made by men for men, but which were presented as applying to everybody. As such, it can be argued that the ideological notion of patriarchy enabled the social control of women by men through language, law, employment and educational opportunities. This led to the discrimination of women that in turn led to their unethical and unfair treatment, which in turn resulted in many women feeling frustrated and oppressed. Those women who were politically active organized themselves into what is known as the suffragette movement that heralded the struggle for the emancipation of women (see Figure 10.1).

Discrimination and oppression operate at both overt and covert levels. Overt discrimination by its very nature is transparent. An example of overt discrimination may be a policy that prohibits same sex couples from sharing a room in a care home. Owing to its transparency, it is easier to address and is often challenged through legislation and policy; for example, the Equality Act 2006 that makes it unlawful to discriminate on the basis of sexual orientation. Covert discrimination on the other hand is much harder to address largely due to its hidden nature, as it is often linked to personal beliefs and values at an unconscious level. Therefore, while discrimination on the basis of sexual orientation is unlawful, people who are gay or lesbians may still experience discrimination due to the homophobic views of individual practitioners (covert discrimination).

Processes of discrimination

In order to understand how and why discrimination occurs, an understanding of the ways in which people can discriminate against others is required. Thompson (2003: 83) refers to these as 'processes of oppression' (Figure 10.2). Essentially, people are discriminated against on the basis of a variety of factors. Most typically it is because they belong to a particular group in society based on, for example, race, sexuality or gender. As a result of belonging to a group, people discriminate against them in a variety of ways (coined by Thompson as the 'processes of oppression'), which results in oppressive language, behaviour and practice. For example, black youths are typically perceived (or stereotyped) as aggressive and involved in gang crime. This can lead to racism. It is important to recognize that the processes of oppression often do not operate in isolation as they frequently interact, combine and reinforce one another.

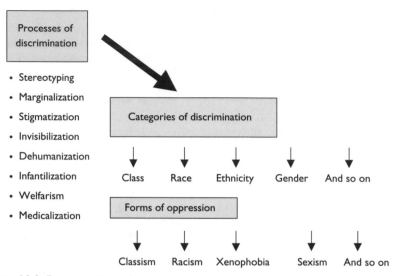

Figure 10.2 Discrimination and oppression
Source: Thompson (2003)

↻ **Activity 10.4 Reflective question**

From your current understanding, try to define the following terms and give examples from your practice experience:

- stereotyping
- marginalization
- stigmatization
- invisibilization
- dehumanization
- infantilization
- welfarism
- medicalization.

Compare your answers with the information contained in the following section.

Stereotyping

Judging people on the basis of the assumptions we hold about them is called stereotyping. These judgements are predicated on the belief that all members within a social group are essentially the same. This leads to unfair and detrimental generalizations about individuals. We may be unaware that we hold these beliefs that prevent us from responding to the uniqueness and individuality of each person. An example of stereotyping is the perception of homosexual men during the 1980s at the time of the outbreak of the

HIV virus and AIDS in the USA and Europe, in that individuals were perceived to be promiscuous and to have multiple sexual partners. This stereotype was further perpetuated in the media at the time and resulted in not only incorrect messages regarding transmission of HIV, but also the assumption that all gay men are promiscuous.

Marginalization

Marginalization occurs when certain groups of people are treated as insignificant and peripheral to society and are thus excluded from mainstream activities. Many people with disabilities have experiences of this process. The DoH (2001a) document *Valuing People* stresses the need for people with disabilities to lead more inclusive lives, in which they feel valued members of society. Yet it can be argued that they are often marginalized and excluded as they are denied opportunities to engage in paid employment (Roulstone and Warren, 2006). They also experience increased levels of unemployment than the general population, and are paid less then their non-disabled counterparts. In addition, the Equality and Human Rights Commission (2008) revealed that there appears to be a culture of low expectation with respect to the opportunities for people with disability, even though there is clear legislation prohibiting discrimination on the basis of disability (Disability Discrimination Act 2005). In addition to economic and employment difficulties, Melville (2005) notes that barriers to accessing health care services also exist that can further perpetuate the inequity that people with disabilities face.

Stigmatization

Stigmatization refers to the process of social relations that lead to and reproduce definitions of 'outsider' and 'others'. Such processes serve to define and label specific groups as being undesirable and dangerous (Goffman, 1963 cited Takahashi, 1997). Green et al. (2003) acknowledge that stigmatization of mental illness is well documented within the nursing literature, for example, stemming from a perception that clients with mental illness are dangerous and unpredictable and that they should be avoided. This view is also perpetuated in the media and has resulted in mental illness being stigmatized within society. Behaviour indicative of mental distress also frequently meets with disapproval and fear.

Invisibilization

Invisibilization refers specifically to how certain groups are represented in language and imagery in a variety of media, films and the arts. More dominant groups, such as heterosexual, white people, for example, are more likely to be represented in various different contexts and situations, while minority groups feature very rarely and when they do this is often with negative connotations. Examples include stereotypical representations of the young, black criminal or the promiscuous gay man. Thus, minority groups are rendered invisible. In health care, for example, sexuality of older people is a neglected issue, perhaps reflecting stereotypical assumptions that older people are asexual. It is perhaps unsurprising therefore that the experience of older gay and lesbians are ignored from a policy, practice and research perspective (Price, 2005). This lack of understanding and attention to issues affecting older gays and lesbians has implications for service provision: for example, a lack of recognition that a same sex partner has next-of-kin status, or their participation in end-of-life care. Thus, the invisibilization of older gays and lesbians has resulted in discrimination in both health and social care contexts as well as within the gay and lesbian community (Ward et al., 2008). One of the implications of invisibilization may be that some older people may feel forced to deny their sexuality.

Dehumanization

This process refers to the ways in which people are stripped of their human attributes and qualities. For example, it could be argued that this can occur during the process of hospitalization as clients' clothes and personal belongings are removed and they lose their individuality and become *patients*. This is further perpetuated with terms such as 'bed blockers', 'the old', and 'the stroke in bed 10', all of which result in the depersonalization of the individual who is referred to. Indeed, the recent report *Seeing the Patient in the Person* (The King's Fund, 2008) challenges that the NHS has to see the person rather than a patient.

Infantilization

Infantilization is the process by which clients are ascribed a child-like status and examples of this could be the language used by some practitioners to older people; for example, 'chicken', 'honey' and 'dear'. Infantilization occurs when there is a mismatch between an individual's ability to communicate and others' perception of that ability (Brown and Draper, 2003). In the case of older people, this is reinforced by negative perceptions and stereotypes in which ageing is associated with mental decline resulting in practitioners using patronizing and inappropriate terms of address.

Welfarism/medicalization

Welfarism relates to a tendency to assume that individuals require welfare services on the basis of belonging to a certain group. Typical examples of this include older people and people with disabilities who are perceived to be unable to live independently or exercise their autonomy. Welfarism can lead to practitioners taking a paternalistic role in client interaction resulting in clients' disempowerment. The process of medicalization works in a similar disempowering way. In this context it usually refers to the attribution of a medical diagnosis to a particular entirely understandable and human state such as distress, for example. So instead of recognizing that somebody is upset and providing comfort, professionals may label them 'psychotic' or 'depressed' and prescribe drugs.

Some of the difficulties regarding the processes of oppression are related to the tendency to group things together. Indeed, this phenomenon is well studied within social psychology and is arguably reinforced by health and social care provision that groups people into categories (e.g. child, adult, mental health and learning disability services). However, it must be recognized that within each group there are multiple individuals, each with differing needs and aspirations. For example, it is often assumed that all older people are the same and have the same needs and interests; however, within the bracket of older people services are a variety of different people with an age span between 65–105 years and beyond. It is therefore important for practitioners to recognize that groups are not homogenous in nature; in addition, it also needs to be acknowledged that multiple oppressions can and does occur; for example, a black older woman who suffers with depression could be oppressed due to the nature of her age, gender, ethnic origin and ongoing health needs.

A model to explore discrimination and oppression

In order to develop an understanding of discrimination and the resulting oppression arising from it, Thompson (2003) argues that it is important to recognize that it operates at three separate, but interrelated levels including the personal, cultural and structural. The case study below serves to illustrate all three levels.

Case study 10.1 Raising awareness

Mary is 78 and has been brought to the local A&E department following a fall; she is unable to weight bear and is accompanied by her husband. The department is very busy; as a result of this Mary is being nursed in the corridor and is awaiting an X-ray. Mary's husband approaches a student nurse because Mary needs to go to the toilet; the student approaches a staff nurse for assistance to move Mary to somewhere more private. The staff nurse informs the student 'there is no where to take her – tell her to wet herself'.

Personal level

Individuals' thoughts, feelings and actions at an individual level can have a major bearing on inequality and oppression. This occurs especially if one individual has greater power over another – in the case study it can be argued that the staff nurse was in a position of power over Mary and may have had negative perceptions regarding older people resulting in oppression occurring at a personal level. This could have occurred through the processes of stereotyping (all older people are incontinent), medicalization (in seeing the disease and losing sight of the person) or dehumanization (removing Mary's clothes and ascribing a medical diagnosis assists in rendering Mary as a disease rather than a person). In addition, the personal level includes the actual experiences of users and in the case of Mary it could be questioned whether she received quality care based on her individual needs or whether the staff attitudes towards her were influenced by a negative perception or stereotype of older people, resulting in poor quality of care being provided and fundamental care needs unmet.

Cultural level

It is important however to remember that individual beliefs are influenced by the surrounding culture. With regard to Mary, the culture of a department that may focus on urgent and emergency care aimed at saving lives may influence the extent to which fundamental care is valued and therefore provided. In addition, cultural values are often transmitted through humour; in Western society age has a very negative view seen as a period of decline often ridiculed in birthday cards, which can influence staff perceptions that it is acceptable to expect an older person to be incontinent. Finally, at the cultural level, the use of language often transmits derogatory and discriminating views from one generation to another; in the case of older people terms such as being 'senile' and having a 'senile moment' that are often used within society could further perpetuate a view of old age being associated with mental decline, therefore Mary would not mind being incontinent of urine. The difficulty with cultural levels of oppression is that like stereotypes individuals are often not aware or challenge these cultural norms resulting in passive oppression.

Structural level

Structural level oppression consists of macro-level influences as well as social, political and economic constraints. In the case of Mary, it can be argued that the unit did not have sufficient capacity to care for the numbers of clients they were presented with, which resulted in clients being nursed in corridors with inadequate levels of privacy. In addition, the extent to which service users and clients are truly involved in the development or review of services needs to be questioned.

Thompson (2003) argues that in challenging oppressive practice, there is essentially no middle ground in that practitioners are either part of the solution or part of the problem. In addition, if we recognize that oppression occurs at three distinct, but interconnected levels, then surely anti-oppressive practice also needs to reflect the personal, cultural and structural levels. Structural levels of oppression are often challenged through laws and policies. In the case of Mary, the *National Service Framework for Older People* (DoH, 2001b) was developed in recognition that there were poor, unresponsive and insensitive services. As such one of its core themes was challenging discriminatory practice. It also clearly stated that discrimination has no place in health services. Yet Age Concern (2008) argue that covert discrimination (as in the case of Mary) still exists in health and social care and that this is due to the fact that structural levels do little to challenge cultural and personal levels of oppression. More recent policy documents such as the *Confidence in Caring* report (DoH 2008b) appear to have incorporated a balance between the three levels insofar as it identifies that caring is not just about what each member of staff does (reflective of the personal level), but also involves the environment, culture, history of the environment and the team (reflective of cultural and structural elements), and the way in which staff behave and interact with each other, patients and their families (personal and cultural levels). Furthermore, the report also identified that all these aspects of care are interdependent and to be effective, change has to be embedded in the whole system and not just one part of it. At a structural or organization level, confidence depends on the means by which care is provided, and this includes the physical features of the clinical area, resources available and the overall culture that is vital to patients. At a cultural or team level, client confidence depends on the way care is delivered, coordinated and led. Finally, at the patient or individual level, confidence is created when clients see that practitioners have the skills to do the job and the will to provide the level of care the client wants.

⟲ Activity 10.5 Reflective Exercise

For each level identified below, critically reflect on your area of practice and identify factors that enhance or hinder the promotion of equality and diversity.

- structural or organizational
- cultural or team
- patient or individual.

Conclusion

Oppression or oppressive practice, even if it is done at an unconscious level, undermines people's ability to participate in health and social care decisions, damages their self-determination and self-esteem and perpetuates social inequalities. It constitutes the exact opposite to empowerment and service user participation and often leads to negative self-perceptions of not being deserving of more resources or increased participation (Prilleltensky and Gonick, 1996). In order to promote equality and diversity in practice development in health and social care, we need to develop an awareness of how the processes of discrimination and oppression work in practice in order to challenge them at personal, cultural and structural levels. By being aware of these mechanisms, we also have more freedom to choose how we respond to others, either as unique individuals or as bearers of particular traits and characteristics belonging to a particular category. The former is more likely to ensure that individuals are at the centre of decision-making and feel empowered to voice their needs while it is also more likely that professionals practising in that way keep their own humanity intact.

We close with a number of key questions that can be used to stimulate thinking both individually and within your area of practice (adapted from Williams, 1999 cited in Chahal, 2006 and Commission for Racial Equality, 2003).

- Do you understand the needs of the diverse group of clients that you care for?
- Do your services meet the diverse needs and aspirations of clients in your care?
- Does your service achieve equally high outcomes for all?
- How can you best keep this situation under review, and continue to monitor impact?
- How can you make clear, both internally and externally, what you are doing?
- What changes can be made that will improve this position?
- What specific outcomes or targets should we be aiming for?

Key points

- Recent legislation and policy to eliminate prejudice, oppression and unlawful, overt discrimination has been an important vehicle for ensuring that the human rights of everyone are respected.
- These laws and guidelines signify a shift of emphasis away from simply outlawing discrimination to the positive duty to promote equality, but covert discrimination is more difficult to tackle.
- Being discriminated against leads to poor mental and physical health.
- The vision of an inclusive and human rights-based approach to policy making, workforce planning and staffing, service commissioning and delivery, inclusive planning and public health strategy has set the tone for the development of practice.
- Discrimination and oppression operate via a number of different processes, such as stereotyping, marginalization, invisibilization, stigmatization, infantilization, and so on and at personal, cultural and structural level. An understanding of these mechanisms is important in challenging discriminatory practices and policies.

Further reading

Jones, L. (1994) *The Social Context of Health and Health Work*. London: Macmillan.
Kelleher, D. (1996) A defence of the use of the terms 'ethnicity' and 'culture', in D. Kelleher and S. Hillier (eds) *Researching Cultural Differences in Health*. London: Routledge.
Northway, R. (1997) Disability and oppression: some implications for nurses and nursing, *Journal of Advanced Nursing*, 26(4): 736–43.
Nzira, V. and Williams, P. (2009) *Anti-oppressive Practice in Health and Social Care*. London: Sage Publications.

Useful links

Equality and Human Rights Commission. Available online at www.equality humanrights.com.
Department of Health Equality and Human Rights section. Available online at www.dh.gov.uk/en/Managingyourorganisation/Equalityandhumanrights/ DH_076743.

References

Age Concern (2008) *Quality not Inequality*. London: Age Concern.
Ashkam, J. (2008) *Health and Care Services for Older People*. London: Department of Health (DoH).
Brown, A. and Draper, P. (2003) Accommodative speech and terms of endearment: elements of a language mode often experienced by older adults, *Journal of Advanced Nursing*, 41(1): 15–21.
Chahal, K. (2006) Discrimination, service provision and minority ethnic user views, *Housing, Care and Support*, 9(1): 25–8.
Commission for Racial Equality (2003) *Towards Racial Equality: An Evaluation of the Public Duty to Promote Race Equality and Good Race Relations in England and Wales*. London: Commission for Racial Equality.
Department of Health (DoH) (2000) *The Vital Connection: An Equalities Framework for the NHS*. London: DoH.
Department of Health (DoH) (2001a) *Valuing People: A new Strategy for Learning Disability for the 21st Century*. London: DoH.
Department of Health (DoH) (2001b) *National Service Framework for Older People*. London: DoH.
Department of Health (DoH) (2008a) *High Quality Care for All (Darzi Report)*. London: DoH.
Department of Health (DoH) (2008b) *Confidence in Caring*. London: DoH.
Department of Health (DoH) and British Institute of Human Rights (2008) *Human Rights in Healthcare: A Framework for Local Action*. London: DoH.
Douglas, D. (2004) Ethical challenges of an increasingly diverse workforce: the paradox of change, *Human Resource Development International*, 7(2): 197–210.
Equality and Human Rights Commission (2008) Response of the Equality and Human Rights Commission to the Office of Disability Issues Consultation 'Improving Protection for Disability Discrimination'. London: Equality and Human Rights Commission.

Fairclough, N. (2003) Political correctness: the politics of culture and language, *Discourse and Society*, 14(1): 17–28.

Green, G., Hayes, C., Dickinson, D., Whittaker, A. and Gilheany, B. (2003) A mental health service users perspective to stigmatisation, *Journal of Mental Health*, 12(3): 223–4.

Hall, P.A. (1999) Social capital in Britain, *British Journal of Political Science*, 29: 417–61.

Health Professions Council (2004) *Standards of Conduct, Performance and Ethics*. London: Health Professions Council.

Hunt, B. (2004) Recent equality legislation in the UK, *Nursing Ethics*, 11: 411–13.

McCormack, B., Manley, K., Titchen, A., Kitson, A. and Harvey, G. (1999) Towards practice development: a vision in reality or a reality without vision, *Journal of Nursing Management*, 7: 255–64.

McSherry, R. and Warr, J. (2008) *An Introduction to Excellence in Practice Development in Health and Social Care*. Maidenhead: Open University Press.

Melville, C. (2005) Discrimination and health inequalities experienced by disabled people, *Medical Education*, 39: 122–6.

Nursing and Midwifery Council (2008) *Code of Conduct for Nurses and Midwives*. London: Nursing and Midwifery Council.

Price, E. (2005) All but invisible: older gay men and lesbians, *Nursing Older People*, 17(4): 16–18.

Prilleltensky, I. and Gonick, L. (1996) Polities change, oppression remains: on the psychology and politics of oppression, *Political Psychology*, 17: 127–47.

Roulstone, A. and Warren, J. (2006) Applying a barriers approach to monitoring disabled people's employment: implications for the Disability Discrimination Act 2005, *Disability and Society*, 21(2): 115–31.

Takahashi, L. (1997) The socio-spatial stigmatization of homelessness and HIV/AIDS: toward an explanation of the NIMBY syndrome, *Social Science of Medicine*, 45(6): 903–14.

The King's Fund (2008) *Seeing the Person in the Patient*. London: The King's Fund.

Thompson, N. (2001) *Anti-discriminatory Practice*, 3rd edn. Basingstoke: Palgrave Macmillan.

Thompson, N. (2003) *Promoting Equality: Challenging Discrimination and Oppression*. Basingstoke: Palgrave Macmillan.

Walsh, K. and Moss, C. (2007) Practice development in New Zealand: reflections on the influence of culture and context, *Practice Development in Health Care*, 6(1): 82–5.

Ward, R., River, L. and Fenge, L. (2008) Neither silent nor invisible: a comparison of two participative projects involving older lesbians and gay men in the United Kingdom, *Journal of Gay & Lesbian Social Services*, 20(1/2): 147–65.

Young, I. (1990) *Justice and the Politics of Difference*. Princeton, NJ: Princeton University Press.

Conclusion: the future facing working in organizations in health and social care

11

Rob McSherry and Jerry Warr

Introduction

As outlined in the Introduction, the aim of this book is to explore and detail the key issues and factors that influence the workings of an organization and how these can be addressed through creating a vision, sharing the vision, collaboration, integrated teamworking and by adopting a person-centred approach to care. This concluding chapter offers a review of the content of the book from three perspectives working in organizations, user-focused care and collaborative working, identifying the key issues and recommendations proposed from each chapter.

Figure 11.1 illustrates the three dimensions that aid excellence in organizational practice development. Each dimension is summarized below, emphasizing the focus taken within each chapter of the book.

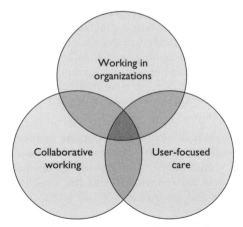

Figure 11.1 The integrated elements of organizational excellence

From these three elements, a framework of considerations has been proposed to support health and social care individuals, teams and organizations to apply, adopt and adapt in the pursing of excellence in practice development associated with working in organizations. It is also viewed as the basis for the future working of health and social care as it becomes increasingly influenced by the commissioning and care quality commission agendas.

Working in organizations: the importance of shared vision

Shared vision is critical to creating cultural change within an organization. It does, however, need to be an achievable, imagined concept of how an organization should (and could) look. It requires leadership and leaders must help their team to create a shared vision that encompasses the goals, values and cultural beliefs of the vision's followers. The followers must recognize the need for change and be involved in the process as failing to create shared vision can incite resistance and coercion. Effective communication is pivotal to unlocking the shared vision and this can be achieved through both language and symbols and through formal and informal methods. The source, message, channel, receiver (SMCR) model provides a useful guide to key aspects of communication. The vision must be inspiring, meaningful and memorable and once developed is best communicated visually. To ensure its acceptance and adoption, consideration must also be given to individual 'conceptual filters'; that is, the ways in which individuals perceive, interpret and adapt information. Finally, creating vision is a continual process.

The role of leadership and change management

Leadership and, in particular, the styles adopted will always be a major determinant in the success or failure of managing change. Although this focuses on the catalyst or primary mover, all staff will have a role to play in shaping and leading service delivery. Innovation and change, problem identification and resolution, quality, performance, outcome(s) and excellence are dependent on how individuals and teams integrate and interact efficiently and effectively as part of the workings of the collective/combined organization.

Leadership qualities are not all innate and should be continually developed and evaluated, positive change, however, cannot take place without emotional commitment. This can be quite challenging and threatening to teams and their members and the organizational culture should foster openness and transparency at all levels, as well as promoting models of inclusiveness.

A whole systems approach

A whole systems approach aims to provide an alternative approach to viewing problems and answering questions. The popularity of systems theory has entered the health and social care arena, in the quest to resolve complex health and social care problems, in an attempt to improve the quality of care and services for patients. As such, it provides an alternative to reductionism, through expansionism, which concentrates on understanding the function and behaviour of the whole system, as opposed to its separate parts. The ultimate goal of whole systems theory is directed towards demonstrating performance in production and output of the organization. Whole systems approaches in the health and social care can be classified, broadly, into three areas: organizational development and service improvement initiatives, quality and performance, and educational and professional developments. Systems can also be classified into two types, hard and soft. Whole systems approaches offer a fantastic opportunity for enhancing the workings of an organization in the quest for quality and excellence.

Collaborative working: cross-professional working

The involvement of all professions and disciplines is a key factor in organizational excellence but collaboration and joint working are vital ingredients. There are obvious benefits to cross-professional/agency working and learning but the benefits, and ways of maximizing vary by the purpose and context of each individual team; thus, there is a need for open and focused dialogue and understanding. There are challenges to cross-professional/agency working including poor inter-professional stereotyping and it is important for practitioners to clarify and clearly articulate their practice, including that part of their practice that involves cross-professional or cross-agency working. The use of activity and social capital theories are tools that practitioners may find useful in this process and have been shown to enhance and develop collaborative, cross-professional working that enhances the client experience and fosters a culture of excellence in practice.

Integrated teamworking

As has been shown above, high-quality health and social care depends on health, social and primary care professionals working and communicating effectively together; it is no more complex than that nor should it be. Since the early 2000s the United Kingdom (UK) health and social care systems have witnessed the introduction of a wide range and diverse set of major government policies advocating integrated teamworking. The drivers for integrated teamworking arise from a vast and varied combination of political, professional and societal factors. It is imperative that health and social care professionals understand the what, why and how integrated teamworking can support enhancing the workings of the organization. Integrated team-working could be summarized as 'the joint working of health and social care professionals to ensure the provision of accessible, seamless services for people when required'. The success of teamworking is the establishment of a recipe for your team and/or organization so that it can be replicated and repeated by anyone with a degree of capability, but that which will guarantee a quality product each time. Offering quality patient-related outcomes associated with integrated teamworking are dependent on awareness raising, sharing, implementation and evaluation of core values. The core values associated with integrated teamworking are a combination and harmonization of having a vision, sharing the vision, encouraging involvement, supporting innovation and change, enthusiasm, communication, collaboration and celebration.

Enabling collaborative working

The enablers and inhibitors to collaborative working can be classified as internal and external factors attributed to individuals or organizations. These are readily themed into seven key headings for which strategies require development in resolving their impact at an organization, team and individual level: culture, management, leadership, communication, education and training, knowledge and support. Management, leadership styles and culture are three enablers and inhibitors that cannot be overlooked from either an organization, team or individual level when considering the implementation of clinical governance. As such a closer inspection of the enabling and inhibiting factors will offer positive and constructive ways of achieving clinical governance provided that adequate support is provided. Education and training for staff on clinical governance is an essential part of collaborative working within an open and no-blame environment. This works best where the user experience is central to care provision and can only be satisfactorily achieved through effective user involvement.

User-focused care: making user involvement a reality

Working in partnership with users of services/patients/carers can be seen to operate on a continuum, from low level involvement through consultative processes through to user-driven developments at the other end of the continuum. Despite the potential benefits of involving users of services/patients/carers in practice development, it is imperative that individuals, teams and organizations understand that adopting participative approaches can sometimes mean that certain disadvantaged groups become further silenced by political disempowerment. Working in partnership with users of services/patients/carers demands trust, time commitment and funding. In practice these issues can prove challenging, particularly issues associated with payments.

Ethical issues in user involvement

User involvement can be conceived as either a 'means to an end' or as an 'end in itself. The former is essentially target-oriented with the aim of containing costs and promoting efficiency and best practice, whereas in the latter user involvement is valued irrespective of tangible outcomes. User involvement can be seen from an economic perspective as consumer choice or from a socio-political perspective as emancipatory and democratic. The way user involvement is framed will have profound ethical implications for practitioners. Power is an important concept in relation to user involvement. Professionals and service users are traditionally positioned in particular relationships with each other as a result of how they are defined by, for example, in terms of social status and knowledge. The following principles are useful when considering ethical conduct in user involvement clarity and transparency, empowerment, identity, commitment to change, respect, equality and diversity, accountability and theoretical assumptions.

Ways of engaging users

Involving service users in clinical and educational developments should be seen as an opportunity to get the 'expert opinion' on how to shape services. Energy and enthusiasm are needed to build a secure infrastructure that will support service user involvement. Learn lessons from other areas but 'one size fits all' are unlikely to be successful. The service user involvement must reflect the local context and be owned by the collective. Investing time in making resources available will reap rewards. Where face-to-face contact is not possible, there are a range of alternative ways for involving service users, such as DVD and audiotape material, website and narrative accounts. Monitoring of involvement is useful to demonstrate how well the organization is facilitating and embedding service user involvement in the cultural fabric.

Promoting equality and diversity

Discrimination and oppression are known to operate via a number of different processes, such as stereotyping, marginalization, invisibilization, stigmatization, infantilization, and so on and at personal, cultural and structural level. Being discriminated against has also been recognized as leading to poor mental and physical health. The vision of an inclusive and human rights-based approach to policy making, workforce planning and staffing, service commissioning and delivery; inclusive planning and public health strategy has set the tone for the development of practice. In fact, legislation and policy to eliminate prejudice, oppression and unlawful, overt discrimination has been an important vehicle for ensuring that the human rights of everyone are respected. These laws and guidelines signify a shift of emphasis away from simply outlawing discrimination to the positive duty to promote equality, but covert discrimination is more difficult to tackle. An understanding of these mechanisms is important in challenging discriminatory practices and policies and promoting excellence in practice.

Working in organizations in health and social care: a model for looking towards the future

We believe that what has been outlined in this book and summarized above provides a robust framework for present and future organizational development that promotes excellence in practice. The three essential integrated elements ensure that the key to success; that is, people are equally represented and that all perspectives are incorporated. As the context of health and social care changes the model is flexible enough to adapt to innovation and change; for example, as new commissioning arrangements are introduced or external measures of performance such as the Care Quality Commission alter their processes of inspection. If excellence is the real aim for a health or social care service, the way the organization operates will remain a major consideration.

We hope you have enjoyed the book.

Further reading

McSherry, R. and Warr, J. (2008) *Introducing Excellence in Practice Development in Health and Social Care*. Maidenhead: Open University Press.

Index

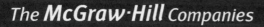
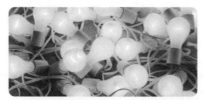 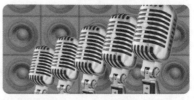
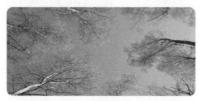 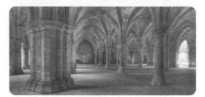
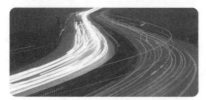 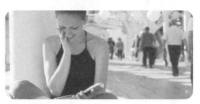
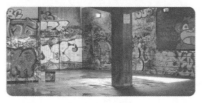
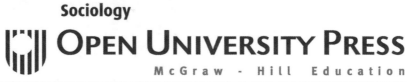